Fatal accidents

Related titles:

Engineering catastrophes: causes and effects of major accidents, third edition
(ISBN 978-1-84569-016-8)
There is much to be gained from the study of catastrophes. Likewise, the records of accidents in industry and transport are of great importance, not only by indicating trends in the incidence of loss or casualties, but also as a measure of human behaviour. The third edition of this well-received book places emphasis on the human factor, with the first two chapters providing a method of analysing the records of accident and all-cause mortality rates to show their relationship with levels of economic development and growth rates, and to make suggestions as to the way in which such processes may be linked.

A quick guide to health and safety
(ISBN 978-1-84569-499-9)
Health and safety issues now impose upon almost every part of business life. The system of enforcement is managed and implemented in the UK by The Health and Safety Executive (HSE) – but at times it can be difficult to know exactly which parts of this elaborate spider's web should be applied in a given instance, and which are most important. This Quick Guide puts the subject into context, providing a rational overview and a valid starting point to applying health and safety in the workplace, and offering a concise and readily accessible interpretation of what health and safety legislation means in practice.

Health and safety in welding and allied processes, fifth edition
(ISBN 978-1-85573-538-5)
The latest edition of *Health and safety in welding and allied processes* has been revised to take into account recent advances in technology and legislative change both in the UK and USA. Beginning with a description of the core safety requirements, it goes on to describe the special hazards found in the welding environment – noise, radiation, fumes, gases – in terms of their effects and the strategies that can be adopted to avoid them. It is an essential resource for welders and their managers.

Details of these and other Woodhead Publishing books can be obtained by:

- visiting our web site at www.woodheadpublishing.com
- contacting Customer Services (e-mail: sales@woodheadpublishing.com; fax: +44 (0) 1223 893694; tel.: +44 (0) 1223 891358 ext. 130; address: Woodhead Publishing Limited, Abington Hall, Granta Park, Great Abington, Cambridge CB21 6AH, UK)

If you would like to receive information on forthcoming titles, please send your address details to: Francis Dodds (address, tel. and fax as above; e-mail: francis.dodds@woodheadpublishing.com). Please confirm which subject areas you are interested in.

Fatal accidents

How prosperity and safety are linked

John Lancaster

CRC Press
Boca Raton Boston New York Washington, DC

WOODHEAD PUBLISHING LIMITED
Oxford Cambridge New Delhi

Published by Woodhead Publishing Limited, Abington Hall, Granta Park, Great Abington, Cambridge CB21 6AH, UK
www.woodheadpublishing.com

Woodhead Publishing India Private Limited, G-2, Vardaan House, 7/28 Ansari Road, Daryaganj, New Delhi – 110002, India

Published in North America by CRC Press LLC, 6000 Broken Sound Parkway, NW, Suite 300, Boca Raton, FL 33487, USA

First published 2009, Woodhead Publishing Limited and CRC Press LLC

British Library Cataloguing in Publication Data
A catalogue record for this book is available from the British Library.

Library of Congress Cataloging in Publication Data
A catalog record for this book is available from the Library of Congress.

Woodhead Publishing ISBN 978-1-84569-530-9 (book)
Woodhead Publishing ISBN 978-1-84569-655-9 (e-book)
CRC Press ISBN 978-1-4200-9483-1
CRC Press order number: WP9483

The publishers' policy is to use permanent paper from mills that operate a sustainable forestry policy, and which has been manufactured from pulp which is processed using acid-free and elemental chlorine-free practices. Furthermore, the publishers ensure that the text paper and cover board used have met acceptable environmental accreditation standards.

Typeset by SNP Best-set Typesetter Ltd., Hong Kong
Printed by TJ International Limited, Padstow, Cornwall, UK

Contents

Preface

While writing a book about engineering catastrophes I decided, for good measure, to include an analysis of fatality rates due to accidents in various industries and modes of transport. The results showed that, with just a few exceptions, these rates declined with the passage of time in a regular, well-ordered fashion.

Whilst this outcome was very satisfactory, it posed some questions: Why the fall? How was it regulated? And why were people (even safety experts) unaware of this improvement in safety?

It was also found that fatal accident rates correlated with economic growth, such that as national output per head increased, the accident mortality rate decreased.

So a model for national progress was set up, in which the development of human skill resulted in higher productivity whilst at the same time the population became more adept at avoiding accidents. Such developments were made possible by progress in science and technology, but the population concerned regulated its pace, and did so subconsciously and collectively. This model was consistent with earlier results, also with data for economic growth and mortality rates from all causes.

The conclusion is that economic growth rates and accident mortality rates are regulated by the population, and that this regulation is accomplished subconsciously.

This conclusion has wide implications, not least for politicians who, in spite of many indications to the contrary, still appear to believe in their power to guide the economy of a country in this way or that.

It is also relevant to government-appointed bodies responsible for legislation on matters pertaining to safety. In the UK, and no doubt in similar developed countries, fatalities due to accidents are falling at a satisfactory rate. Consequently there is no case for legislation, and the activities of such organisations should perhaps be restricted to data collection and analysis.

No call for immediate action, therefore, arises from the present study. There is, however, much scope for further work. Only a very small proportion of the data available worldwide has been examined here. There are many aspects of human behaviour other than the fall in fatal accident rates that may be explored by analysing such data, and if this task be deemed tedious and not compatible with the dignity of human beings, consider the opinion of the poet Alexander Pope:

> Know then thyself, presume not God to scan
> The proper study of mankind is man

Acknowledgements

The author would like to thank the staff of libraries in West Sussex, and in the University of Sussex, for their help; also of the Office for National Statistics, particularly the mortality section, whose compact disc for England and Wales is a notable achievement. Data were also kindly supplied by the Civil Aircraft Authority, Gatwick, Lloyd's Register of Shipping, Marsh and McLennan, Det Norske Veritas, and the Railway Inspectorate, London.

Especial thanks are due to Martin Woodhead and Sheril Leich for rescuing an apparently unpublishable book from oblivion; also to Sarah Green for an excellent typescript.

1 How fatal accidents happen

1.1 Introduction

There is, of course, no generally accepted theory pertaining to accidents. They happen unexpectedly, as a bolt from the blue, and as such, would hardly be expected to fall into any predictable, formal pattern. Least of all would it be expected that we – that is to say the population at large – should regulate the rate at which they occur. Yet analysing the historical records of fatal accidents shows that such is the case: that world-wide their incidence falls into a regular pattern and that, in most types of human activity, the fatal accident rate has fallen during the twentieth century in such a way that it can be represented by a simple mathematical formula.

There is a case, therefore, for seeking a formal model that would be consistent with this pattern of events. Proposals to this end will be made at the end of this chapter. Firstly, however, it is necessary to review some of the evidence. This review will start with an international survey, and then proceed to look at how, in one particular area – England and Wales – the fatal accident rate is affected by age and sex. Finally, road transport deaths in Great Britain (that is to say England, Scotland and Wales) will be subject to a detailed analysis, which in turn will form the basis for the proposed theoretical model.

A list of sources is given in the Appendix. A great deal of the statistical data recorded in this book comes from the records of the English census office, which produced its first annual report in 1841. This document listed the numbers and causes of deaths, and in 1858 the category 'Accident or Negligence' was included. Thus, data for accident mortality in England and Wales are available from this date.

Governments provide information about industry and transport, and a wide variety of organisations maintain information about international activities such as shipping, air transport, the oil industry and so forth.

Methods for analysing data are detailed in Chapter 5. The aim of such analysis is to establish trends, and to determine how accident fatality rates correlate with other measures of human activity, such as national productivity. The results are set out in graphical form, with accident mortality rates plotted vertically and other variables, including time, on the horizontal scale. The basic unit of time is 1 year but some data will be set out at 10-year or other intervals, as may be appropriate.

1.2 International comparisons: natural disasters

Figure 1.1 shows the accident mortality rate (that is: the annual number of deaths due to accidents, divided by the national population in millions) as a function of national prosperity, as indicated by the national output per head expressed in the US dollar equivalent. The solid line shown on the diagram is the curve that best fits the data points shown. It is a hyperbola, and indicates a reciprocal relationship between the accident mortality rate and the national output per head; in other words, accident mortality rates due to natural disasters are lower in the countries with higher productivity.

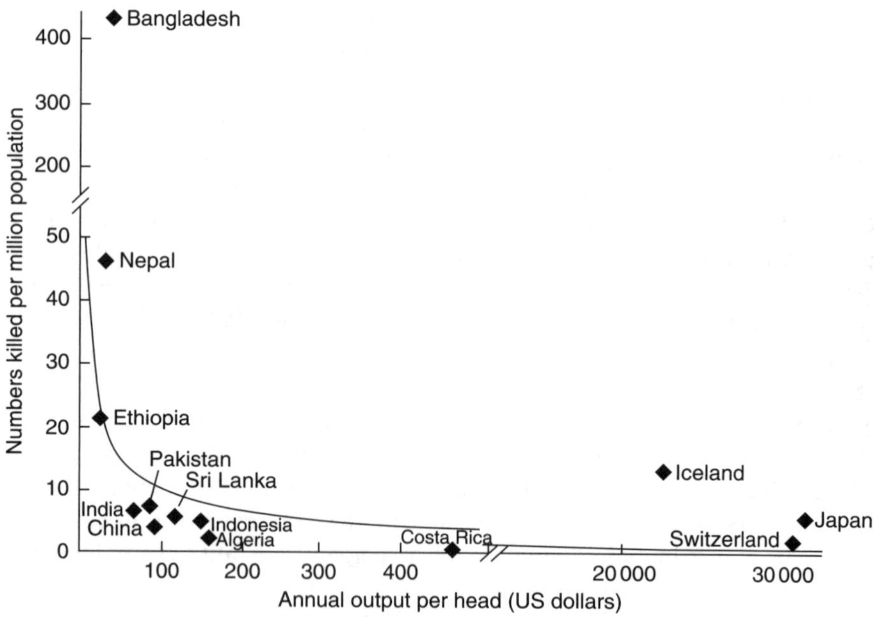

1.1 Annual accident mortality per million population due to natural disasters in various countries as related to the national output per head, expressed in terms of US dollars. Mortality data are from the annual report of the Red Cross, and national output from the United Nations Yearbook. The period is the early 1990s.

Natural forces strike impartially at rich and poor, so at first sight this correlation may appear to be unnatural. Second thoughts indicate otherwise. People belonging to the more prosperous nations have more weather-resistant dwellings and better defences against flood; where earthquakes are prevalent, they have earthquake-resistant buildings and so forth. Avoiding deaths is one of the incentives for human progress, so it is predictable that progress and safety should march together.

1.3 International comparisons: road deaths

Figure 1.2 is similar in character to Fig. 1.1 but, in this instance, relates the annual fatality rate due to road accidents to the national output per head for various countries. The fatality rate is measured as the annual number of road deaths per 10000 registered vehicles. It is assumed that the vehicle numbers provide a good approximation to the size of the driver population, so that the ordinate values in both diagrams are effectively of the same type. The fatality rate is the annual number of deaths per head of the population, although in this instance we are concerned with a sub-population of vehicle drivers instead of the national population.

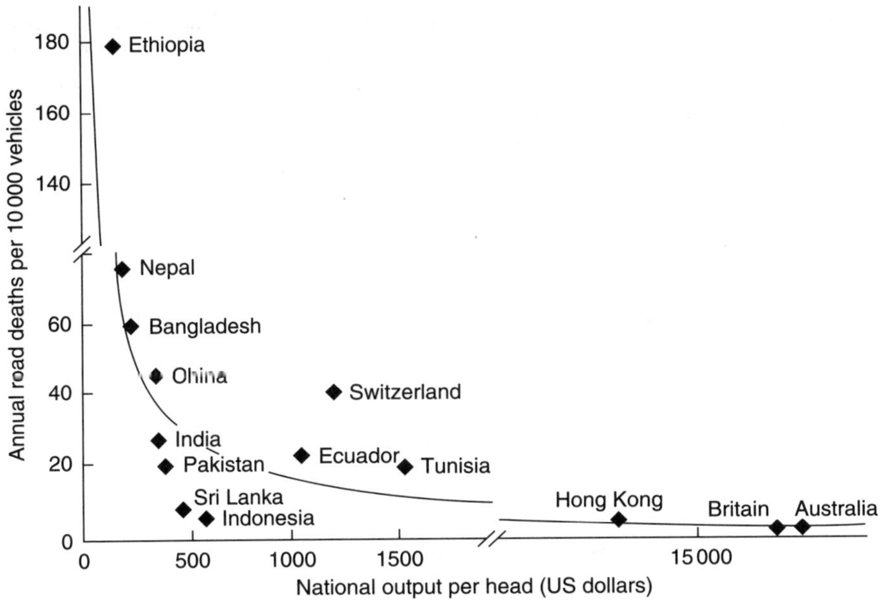

1.2 Relationship between fatality rate in road accidents and national output per head for various countries. The scale is altered at the points indicated in order to accommodate extreme data:sources as for Fig. 1.1.

The units in Figs. 1.1 and 1.2 may be similar, but they relate to very different types of accident. In the first instance, multiple deaths are caused by a single uncontrollable force. In the second, fatalities result from numerous events, most of which are caused by an error of judgement by a single human being. In both cases the relationship with the level of economic progress is similar. The reason why this should be so will be explained later in this chapter.

1.4 Changes in the causes of accidental death

Since accident mortality rates are lower where national productivity is higher, and since national productivity in a given country increases with time, it is reasonable to expect that, in a particular country, accident mortality rates will decrease with time. This is indeed the case, but before exploring this relationship, it will be useful to consider how *causes* of fatal accidents have changed with time.

Figure 1.3 is a bar chart showing the proportion of fatal accidents due to various causes in 1859, and Fig. 1.4 is a similar chart for the year 2000. The most frequent cause in 1859 was 'fractures and contusions' at 42%, and this category has been interpreted as injuries due to falls. The 2000 figure is almost identical at 42.5% and indeed falls (for example, down stairs or from a ladder) are accepted to be the most common cause of accidental death, and here there has been no significant change. Fire remains a major hazard, and transport has replaced 'droving' as the other main cause. The rise of the motorcar population during the twentieth century has had a profound effect on daily life and, as will also be seen elsewhere in this chapter, on the incidence of accidental death.

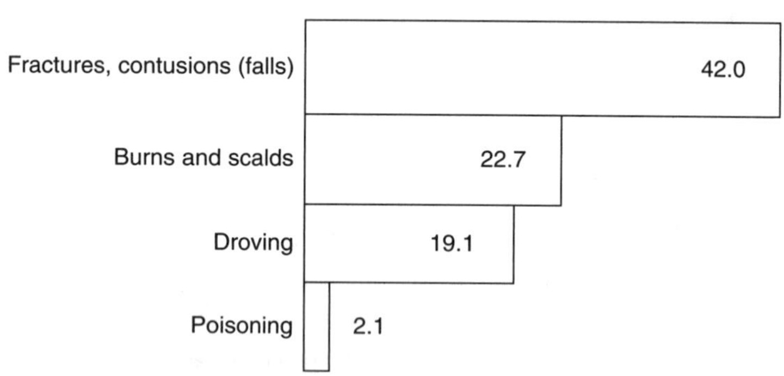

1.3 Causes of accidental deaths in England and Wales for 1859: other causes amounted to 14.1% and included suffocation, gunshot and stab wounds. In this and in Fig. 1.4 the inset figures are the percentage of all accidental deaths.

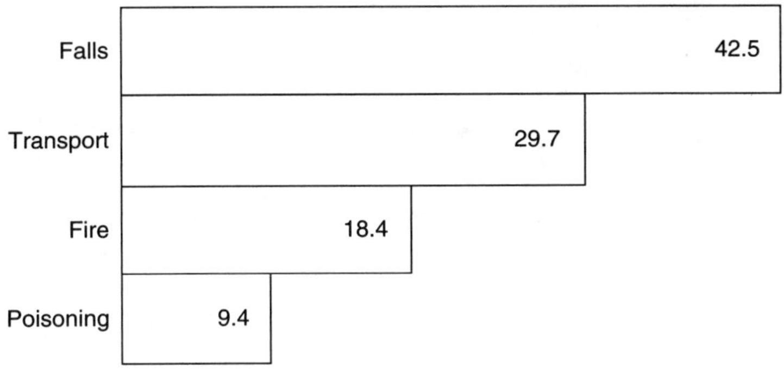

1.4 Causes of accidental deaths in England and Wales for the year 2000.

Another notable change is the increase in the proportion of deaths due to accidental poisoning. This has two main sources. The first, which was operative during the first half of the twentieth century, was carbon monoxide. This poisonous gas was a constituent of town gas and motor vehicle exhausts. Both these hazards have been overcome: the first by changing the domestic gas supply to non-poisonous methane and the second by fitting vehicle exhausts with catalytic converters. The increase in accidental poisoning has been maintained, however, through poisoning by drugs, that is to say through misuse of illegal narcotic drugs, and also by accidental overdoses of medicinally prescribed drugs.

1.5 The accident mortality rate and national productivity

In Fig. 1.5 the accident mortality rate for England and Wales is plotted against the national output per head for Great Britain during the period 1861 to 2000. About 90% of the population of Great Britain lives in England and Wales, so the geographical discrepancy is not significant. Thus, the accident mortality rate does indeed fall with an increase in national prosperity. It would seem reasonable to consider that the increase in national prosperity relates to an increase of skill on the part of the British population, and that, by the same token, this population has become more adept at avoiding accidents. Also, the conditions of a more prosperous life are intrinsically safer: the pavements are more level and so on. Also, it could be that, with the passage of time, the level of acceptable risk declines.

There are two major deviations to be observed in Fig. 1.5. There is a low point for the year 1921, and a relatively high point for 1941. These correspond, respectively, to the economic depression that followed the 1914–1918 war, and to the economic boom years of the Second World War. They

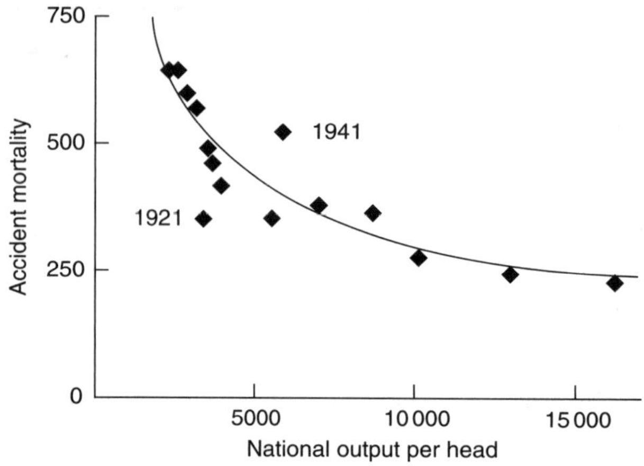

1.5 Relationship between accident mortality per million in England and Wales and annual national output per head for Great Britain. The data points represent individual years at 10-year intervals from 1861 to 2000. The national output is calculated at constant prices in terms of the value of the pound sterling in 2000.

suggest that the correlation between accident mortality and prosperity also applies to temporary deviations in economic growth: accident rates are higher in boom years and lower during periods of slump. This feature will be explored in Chapter 4. But there may be additional or alternative reasons for the upturn in 1941: these are discussed later in this chapter.

1.6 The exponential trend curve

The curves that represent a best fit to the data points in Figs. 1.1 and 1.2 are *hyperbolas*, and are represented by an equation of the form

$$R = a/Q^n \qquad [1.1]$$

where

R is the fatality rate
Q is the national output/head
a and n are constants.

This type of expression is appropriate because the quantities in the denominator of the equation are all *finite*. In plotting fatality rates against time, however, this is no longer the case. Time may extend to an infinite extent ahead of, and behind, the present, and it is necessary to seek an expression that will accommodate this state of affairs. The *exponential* equation

$$R = ae^{bt} \qquad [1.2]$$

satisfies this requirement. In this expression R is the fatality rate, t is the time and a and b are constants. When t is minus infinity, R is zero; when t is infinite, R is also infinite. So, R varies continuously and is always positive. Also, the proportional rate of change of R is constant and equal to b. Thus, if the unit of time is 1 year, the fatality rate changes by the amount bR each year. Actual mortality and fatality rates conform generally with this requirement but the 'constant' b varies slightly with time. In the case of a declining rate, b is negative. Where this is the case, the rate approaches zero as time increases, but always remains finite, however small.

Thus in seeking a trend curve to represent the variation of fatality rates with time, the exponential form will invariably be selected whenever this is appropriate. This is the case for most human activities during the late nineteenth – and for most of the twentieth – century. There are exceptions which will be considered in due course. There remains the question as to what happened before records began. Extrapolating trend curves backwards in time for the recorded period soon produces impossibly high accident mortality rates. It would seem that, in recent times, there has been an increase in both the pace at which accident mortality rates have fallen and national productivity has augmented, and the general correlation established in Figs. 1.1 and 1.2 suggests a slower improvement during previous millennia.

Reference has been made above to 'mortality' and 'fatality' rate. The term 'accident mortality rate' will be used for those instances relating to the whole national population, whilst 'fatality rate' will refer to specific activities, such as the manufacturing industry, where only a proportion of the national population is employed.

1.7 Male and female accident mortality rates

In Fig. 1.6 male and female accident mortality rates for England and Wales have been plotted from 1860 to the year 2000.

The difference between these two plots is a characteristic feature of such comparisons: female accident mortality rates tend to be low and steady whilst male rates deviate upwards. Thus, in 1860 the male accident mortality rate was about three times that for females. Subsequently, in conformity with general trends, both rates have diminished: that for males by about 1% annually, and for females by 0.05%, so that, by the year 2000, the rates were only marginally different.

Accident mortality rates also vary according to age. Figures 1.7 and 1.8 show this variation for the years 1861 and 2000, respectively. In these plots the mortality figures are for age groups. These are 1–4 years, 5–9, 10–14, 15–19, 20–24, and subsequently for 10-year periods, 25–34, etc. The 'median' is the middle figure for the group: thus for 5–9 the median is 7.

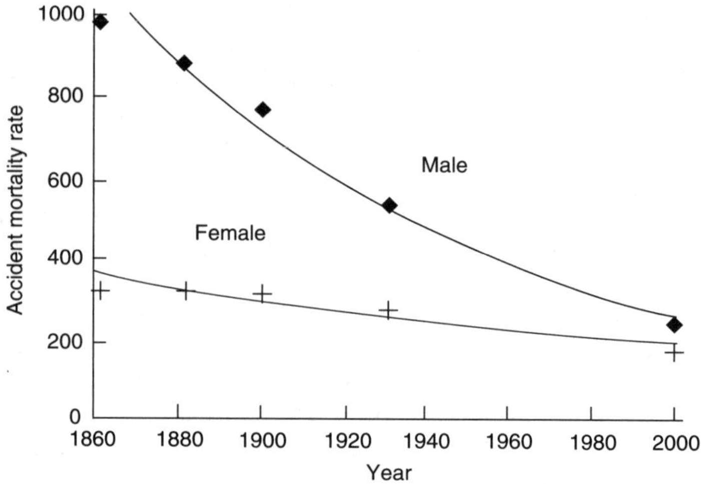

1.6 Annual accident mortality rate per million population according to sex in England and Wales from 1861 to 2000. The rate for males declined at about 1% annually; that for females at about 0.05%.

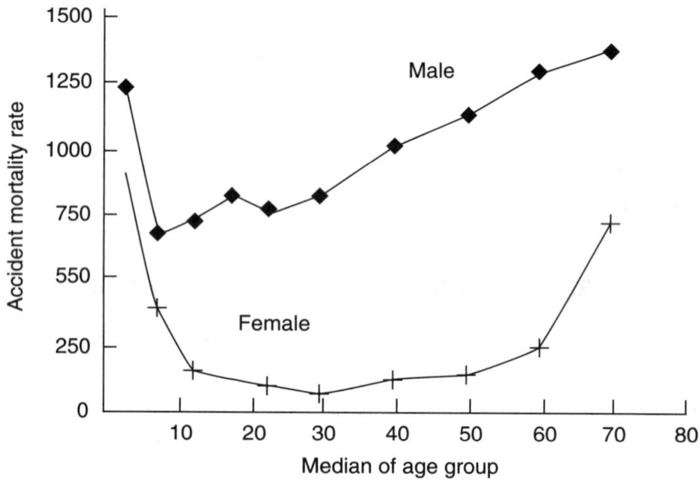

1.7 Annual mortality rate per million population due to accidents in England and Wales in 1861 according to sex and age group.

These two plots are characteristic in that, for very young children, the rates are similar for both sexes, whilst for old persons they once again approach each other. Between these extremes, the female plot generally tends to a U-shaped curve, whilst male rates increase generally with age, but have a peak typically corresponding to the 15–19 or 20–24 age group.

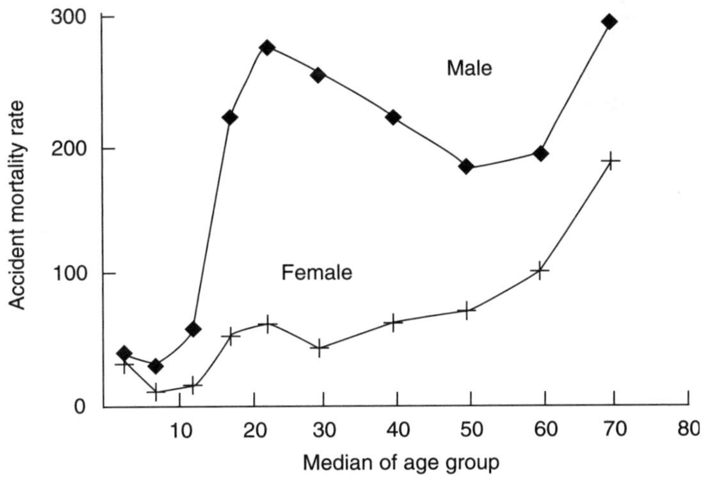

1.8 Annual mortality rate per million population due to accidents in England and Wales in 2000 according to sex and age group.

A notable difference between the plots in Figs. 1.7 and 1.8 is the level of mortality rates for very young children. These fell from about 1000 in 1861 to less than 50 in the year 2000. This must reflect a radical improvement in the standards of care and protection during the period in question.

1.8 Fatal accidents in time of war

It was observed earlier in this chapter that accident mortality rates for civilians in 1941 were significantly higher than the general trend, and this fact was considered to be an effect of the Second World War. Such increases were indeed a feature of both the 1914–1918 and the 1939–1945 wars. They did not occur during any of the localised conflicts – the South African or Korean wars, for example, that took place in the post-1858 period.

In Figs. 1.9 and 1.10 the accident mortality figures for the 40–44 age group are plotted for the two relevant periods. It will be seen that males were entirely responsible for the increased rate, and this was also the case for other adult age groups, although there are some irregularities; in the 20–24 age group, for example, accident mortality rates decreased during the later years of the Second World War. This was probably due to the fall in the numbers and use of motorcars during that time.

It must be emphasised that all accident mortality data considered here pertain to *civilians*, and none relate to any soldiers, sailors or airmen. Thus, it would seem that the threat to national integrity implicit in a world war caused young (and some not so young) civilian men to accept a higher level of risk, and thereby incur a higher rate of fatal accidents.

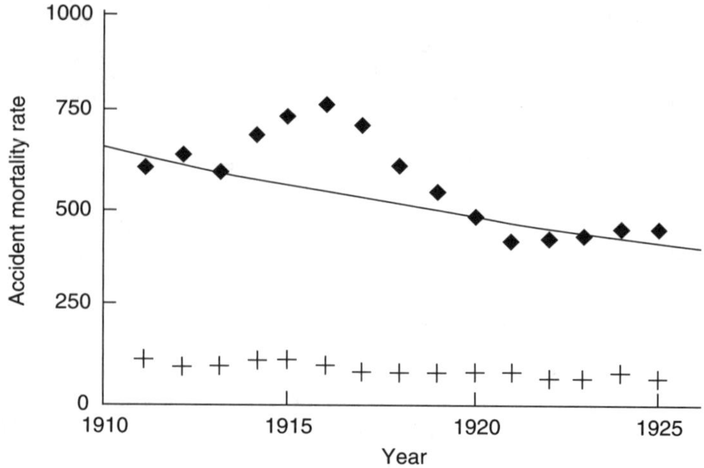

1.9 Annual mortality rate per million population due to accidents in England and Wales 1911–1925 for the age group 40–44. ◆ male; + female.

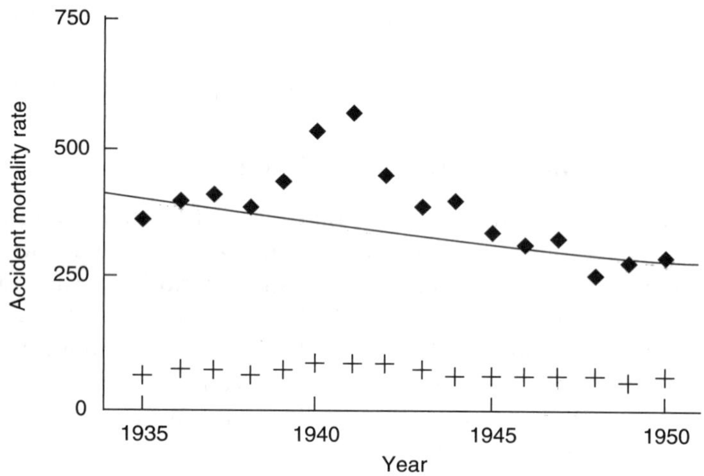

1.10 Annual mortality rate per million population due to accidents in England and Wales 1935–1950 for the age group 40–44. ◆ male; + female.

During the twentieth century, accident mortality rates in general, and those of the 40–44 age group in particular, were declining exponentially, and this has been ascribed here to a development of collective human skill, such that accidents occur at a lower rate. In Figs. 1.9 and 1.10 the solid line indicates the relevant trend curve. Now it will be seen that, in both instances, the data points at the end of the war return to the trend curve, albeit at a lower level than at the beginning of the conflict. It would seem as though some unseen hand is guiding these men back to the 'correct' level of safety.

No such hand exists, however. It is suggested that the wartime upturn of male mortality rates resulted from the actions of a minority of the population in question and that, for the majority, mortality rates continued to decline in the normal manner. Then, when hostilities ceased, the more reckless (or bolder) types conformed with the majority at an improved level of safety.

This explanation implies that the increase in male accident mortality amongst civilians is the result of a change in human behaviour rather than a change in physical circumstances. It might, alternatively, be considered that an increase in fatal accidents is the inevitable result of longer hours and more arduous work in wartime factories. However, it must be remembered that women were recruited in large numbers for factory work during both wars, and that they were exposed to the same physical conditions. There is, however, no evidence in the record, of any increase in accident mortality rates amongst females, as will be evident from Figs. 1.9 and 1.10. Male behaviour in the time of war is not the result of adverse physical condition; on the contrary, it makes its own rules: it is *self-regulating*.

1.9 Fatal accidents on roads in Great Britain

Most of the records presented so far in this chapter have been general in character, being concerned with mortality rates for the whole population, and, most particularly, with the population of England and Wales. In this section it is proposed to review information concerning the fatality rate due to road accidents, with special attention to accidents on roads in Great Britain.

The general relationship between national productivity and fatality rates in road accidents is presented in Fig. 1.2. Great Britain does not feature on this diagram, but it ranks with other developed nations at the right-hand end of the trend curve. The countries of Western Europe and North America have similar records concerning road accident fatality rates and, within the group, Great Britain has one of the lowest fatality rates. These rates will be measured here in the units indicated in Fig. 1.2: namely, annual deaths per 10000 registered vehicles.

Motor vehicles appeared in significant numbers on roads in Europe during the 1920s and, since that time, have caused a substantial proportion of all accidental deaths. Figure 1.11 plots this proportion as a percentage for Great Britain between 1901 and 1985. At the beginning of the century, accidental death on the roads amounted to 10% of all accidental deaths but, with the advent of the motor vehicle, this figure rose to a level which

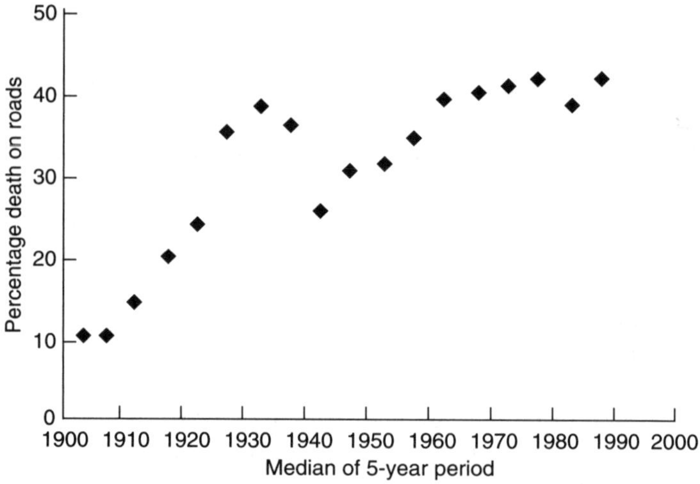

1.11 Percentage of annual accidental deaths resulting from road accidents in Great Britain 1901–1985. Data are 5-year average plotted at the median of the 5-year period.

varied between 25–40%. This situation does not presage a catastrophe: in spite of the rise in the number of motor vehicles and the motorcar in particular, accident mortality rates have fallen during the twentieth century, and there is every expectation that this trend will continue. Nevertheless, the motorcar has had a profound effect on the way of life all over the world, and the relative increase in road deaths is part of this change.

1.10 Road casualties: sex and age

It is common knowledge that the incidence of road accident fatalities varies greatly with sex and age, and that young men are especially at risk. Figure 1.12 shows annual fatalities due to road accidents in Great Britain during 2000 as a percentage of all such fatalities in accordance with sex and age group. It confirms the notion that young men (age group 20–29) are most likely to be so affected. It also shows that, despite the convergence of mortality rates with the passage of time, the difference between males and females in the risk of being killed by accident still persists.

1.11 Road casualties: the normal case

At this stage it is proposed to analyse the historical record of fatal road accidents in Great Britain. Data are provided by the Office for National Statistics, in London, and the record starts in 1926. In general, the figures to be employed are those for all road users and all vehicles, but in some

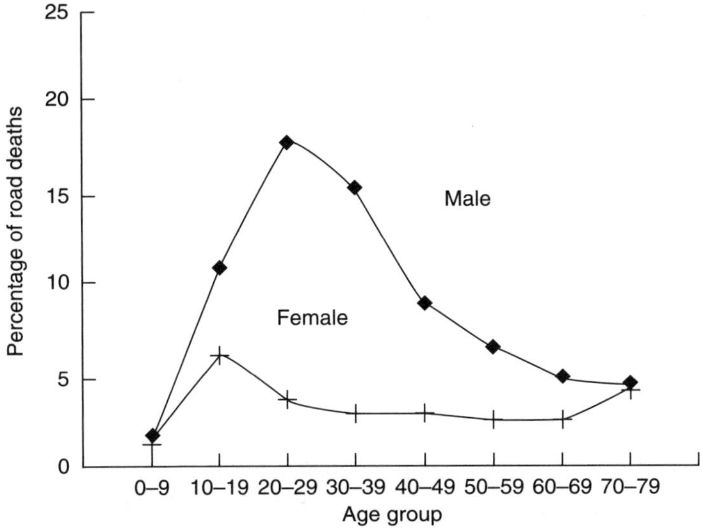

1.12 Percentage of all deaths due to road accidents in Great Britain during 2000 according to sex and age group.

cases it will be necessary to narrow the field: to motorcars, for the effect of the seat belt law, and for motorcycling, which is reviewed in Chapter 2.

This analysis has two main objectives. The record of road casualties shows great regularity, such that the pattern of events provides an archetype for the other activities considered in Chapter 2: in particular, for most of the period under review, the fatality rate declines exponentially with time, and this is considered to be the normal case. Secondly (and this is much more important), the nature of road transport is peculiarly adapted to understanding the way in which self-improvement (in this instance, the reduction of the fatality rate) is accomplished, so that a model of the process can be set up.

The time-dependent record of fatalities due to road accidents in Great Britain falls into two phases. Figure 1.13 is a plot for the first period: that from 1926 to 1934. During this time, fatality rates showed a steadily increasing trend. The solid line in Fig. 1.13 is the best fit to the data points shown. This indicates a modest rate of increase: it also corresponds with the increase in the proportion of deaths due to road accidents as shown in Fig. 1.11.

Figure 1.14 plots road accident fatality rates in Great Britain during the second phase, from 1935 to 2000. The data points indicate a very regular exponential fall in the fatality rates. Data for the war years 1939–1945 have been omitted: these deviate upwards and will be considered later. The solid line is the trend curve corresponding to the data points shown. As before, it follows the equation

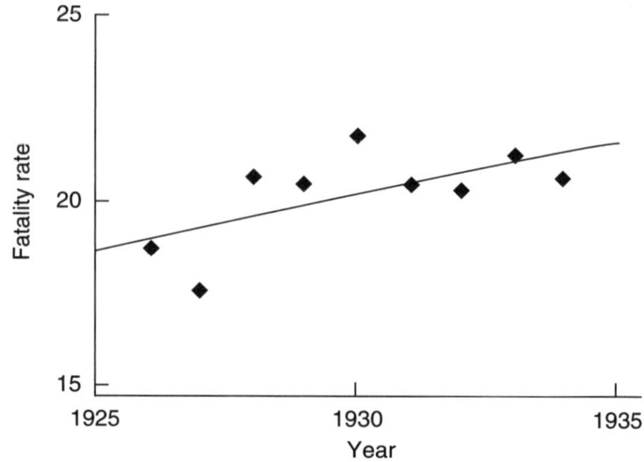

1.13 Annual fatality rate per 10 000 vehicles due to accidents on roads in Great Britain 1926–1934. All road users, all vehicles.

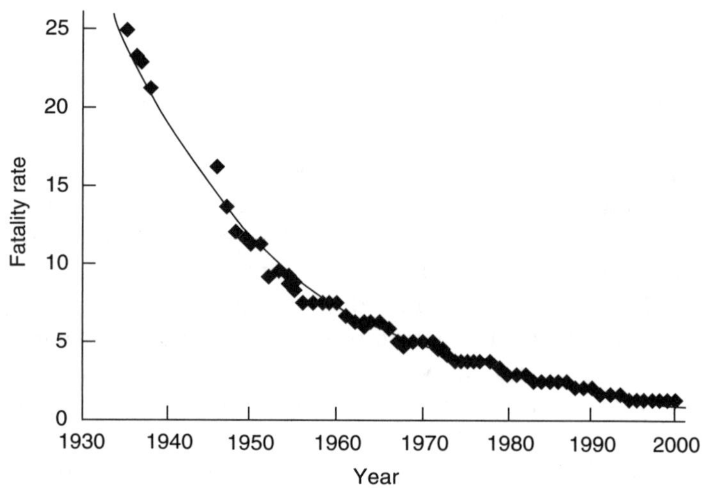

1.14 Annual fatality rate per 10 000 vehicles due to accidents on roads in Great Britain 1935–2000. All road users, all vehicles.

$$R = ae^{bt} \qquad [1.2]$$

where R is the fatality rate, t is time in years, whilst a and b are constants.

This plot, and others of a similar type, have two main characteristic parameters. The first is the constant b, which in the present instance is equal to –0.045. This means that there is a proportional reduction of the fatality rate of 0.045, or 4.5%, per year on average. This is a relatively high figure: the value of *b* for accident mortality and fatality rates during the twentieth century rarely exceeds 6% annually.

It will be evident from the most cursory look at Fig. 1.14 that the road accident fatality data points conform very closely to the trend curve. However, it is possible to be more specific. A measurable quantity known as the *correlation coefficient* determines how well a set of data conforms to a trend. This quantity ranges numerically from 0 to 1; when it is zero, there is no correlation and the data points are scattered entirely at random, but if it equals 1, all data points lie exactly on the trend curve. In the case of Fig. 1.14, the numerical value of the correlation coefficient is 0.9959.

The second characteristic feature of such a set of data points is the degree to which they scatter, relative to the trend curve. Now it is found, in this instance, that the width of the scatter band at any point on the trend curve is proportional to the value of the trend curve at that point: thus the proportional, or relative, width of the scatter band is constant. There is a quantity, the relative standard deviation, from which the width of the scatter band may be calculated (see Chapter 5 for details). This calculation has been made for the road accident fatality rate data and the result, for the period 1971–1990, is shown in Fig. 1.15. If data points conform to a standard model, then 95% of them should fall within a bandwidth equal to four standard deviations. This is indeed the case here.

The significance of these analyses is that fatal road accidents in Britain (and, by implication in other developed countries) are not random, unco-

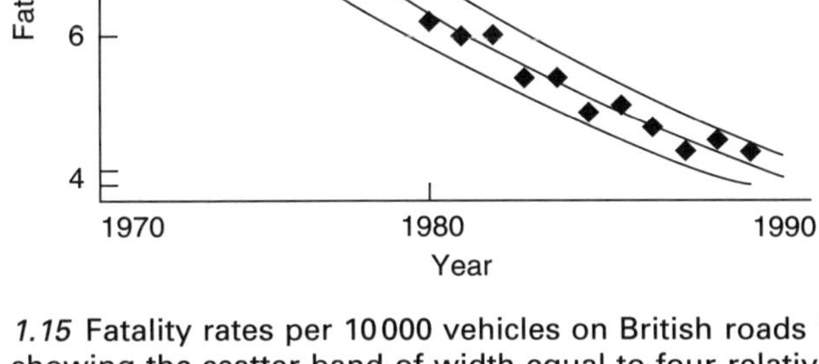

1.15 Fatality rates per 10 000 vehicles on British roads 1971–1990, showing the scatter band of width equal to four relative standard deviations.

ordinated events. On the contrary, they conform to a very regular pattern with respect to time, such that the data can be represented by a simple mathematical model. In other words, these events are regulated, and since there is no external authority capable of such a function, they must be regulated by the population of drivers.

1.12 The effect of the Second World War

Data for the 1939–1945 war were excluded from consideration previously because they were atypical, and Fig. 1.16 shows that this was, indeed, the case. The upward deviation is similar to that for accident mortality in general, but in this instance the rate is calculated per 10 000 vehicles (and, by implication, according to the population of vehicle drivers) rather than the national population, and data are for both sexes and all ages. The return to conformity to the pre-war trend is however particularly evident in this instance. Previous evidence suggests that the upward deviation during the war resulted from the activity of a minority of males, particularly those in the 20–29 age group; that the exponential fall in fatality rates continued during the war amongst the majority of drivers, and in 1946 the minority conformed to the new, lower fatality rate that then prevailed.

As for accident mortality in general, there was no evidence of any increase in road accident fatality rates during local wars.

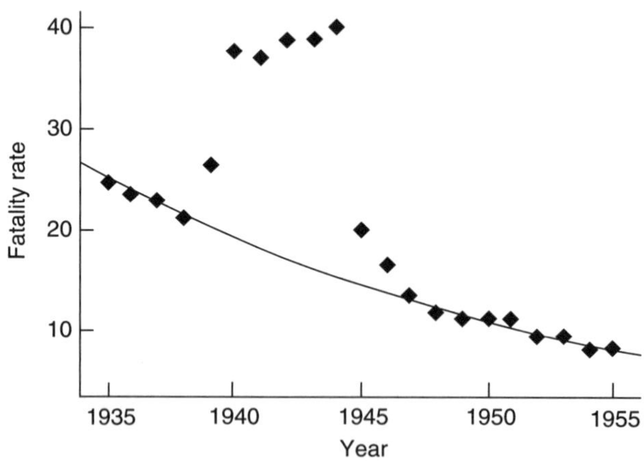

1.16 Annual fatality rates per 10 000 vehicles due to accidents on British roads 1935–1955 for all vehicles and all road users.

1.13 The seat belt law in Great Britain

During the later part of the twentieth century, it became general practice amongst developed nations to require the use of seat belts in motorcars. In Britain this became a legal requirement on 1 February 1983 for the front seat occupants of motorcars and light vans. The law was scheduled to remain in force for a period of three years, at the end of which time the results would be assessed. Government-appointed statisticians reported that the trial had shown that the use of seat belts had indeed reduced casualties, and the law was confirmed. Others, however, examined the same statistics and came to the opposite conclusion.

Trials made with dummies had shown that, in the event of a collision, the wearing of seat belts would greatly reduce the risk of impacts that could cause injury or death. The seat belt law should, therefore, have resulted in a general proportional reduction in the fatality rate, which would, in the plot of such rates against time, have caused a downward displacement of the data points, with a corresponding lowering of the trend curve.

Figure 1.17 is a plot in which data for the ten years prior to 1983 have been plotted together with those for the subsequent ten years, together with the trend curves for the two periods, calculated separately. All data are for the occupants of motorcars.

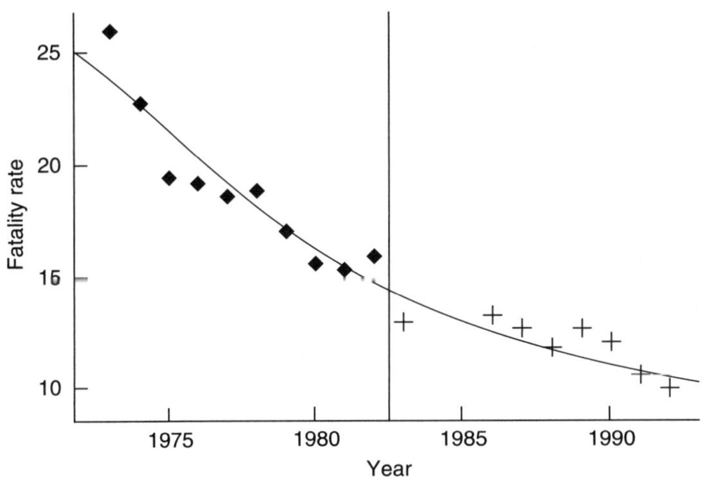

1.17 Annual fatality rate for occupants of motorcars on British roads per 10 000 motorcars, comparing data for the period 1973–1982 with those for 1983–1992. The trend curves shown were calculated separately for the relevant period.

It will be evident that the expected downward displacement after 1983 did not take place, and in particular, that the trend curves meld together almost exactly. The only observable difference is that, after 1983, the fatality rate decreased less rapidly than it did previously.

Others, who have come to similar conclusions about the effect of the seat belt law, have suggested that drivers compensated for the extra security provided by the seat belt by driving more recklessly. Supposing this to be the case, it would be expected that fatality rates of pedestrians should have increased after 1983. This was indeed the case, and a plot of the relevant figures (not reproduced here) for the same two ten-year periods shows an upward displacement of data points and trend curve after 1983. The effect was small, but quite positive.

1.14 The anatomy of self-improvement in accident mortality

It was established at the beginning of this chapter that there exists an inverse relationship between accident fatality and mortality rates and the level of prosperity of individual nations, and it has been shown that, in Great Britain (which is considered here as representative of developed nations) as the national economy grows, so accident mortality rates decrease. It is considered that these correlations are not fortuitous, but that, as the productive skill of a population develops, so does its ability to avoid accidents. Thus, with improvements in engineering, we are better able to resist floods and similar disasters, and improvements in housing and domestic arrangements would be expected to reduce the risk of accidents to children. Also, recalling the fall in male accident mortality shown in Fig. 1.6, it may be that, as standards of personal well-being rise, the level of acceptable risk falls.

To throw some more light on the process that gives rise to a reduction of fatal accident rates, it will be profitable to consider the case of road accident fatality rates in more detail.

It is consistent with previous conclusions that the reduction of fatality rates is the result of a development of skill on the part of the vehicle drivers and other road users. Nowadays, drivers cannot communicate in plain language but must resort to cruder means such as sounding horns, flashing lights or making gestures. It follows that the learning process bears no resemblance to that in a school classroom, but must be more akin to the manner in which an apprentice learns his craft: merely by imitating the master craftsman. Thus, the learning process has three characteristics. Firstly, it occurs through emulation of the skill of other drivers. Secondly, it is, by its nature, collective in character. Thirdly, it occurs as a refinement

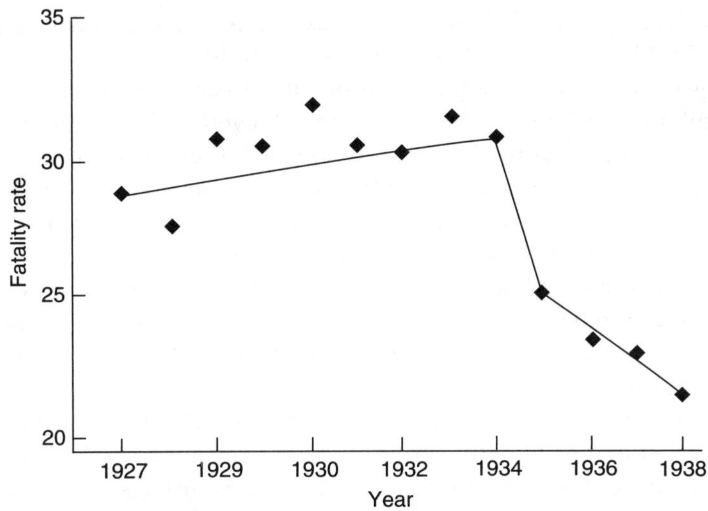

1.18 The transition from a rising fatality rate on British roads to a regulated fall. Data points represent fatality rates per 10000 vehicles 1927–1938.

of judgement; in other words, it results from development in the subconscious part of the brain.

So far as this final proposition is concerned, it is useful to consider the transition from the rising trend of road casualties that occurred in Britain between 1927 and 1934, and the falling trend that has subsequently obtained.

Figure 1.18 is a plot of road accident fatality rates from 1927 to 1938, together with the relevant trend curves. It will be evident that the change from a rising rate to an exponentially falling trend took place abruptly during the year 1935. Now this change could not possibly have resulted from any technical improvement: such changes are gradual both in their introduction and their effect. A driving test became obligatory in Great Britain on 1 June 1935, but this applied to new drivers only, and its physical effect, if any, would have been marginal. The most probable cause of the transition was, therefore, a change in attitude on the part of the driving population as a whole.

In its early days in Great Britain, motoring was a sporting and leisure activity. Sport on the road results in casualties as the contemporary record for motorcycling demonstrates (see Chapter 2). The rising number of road casualties was generally considered to be unacceptable, and made frequent newspaper headlines. So, there was a good deal of moral pressure, and it may be that the forthcoming driving test was an additional stimulus. Whatever the cause, the outlook of drivers changed to one that favoured greater safety. No instructions to this effect were given, however, and nobody at the time noticed or recorded change. It was previously regulated, as was the exponential fall of the fatality rates that followed.

Following this train of thought, it is possible to envisage a means by which the regulation of fatality rates could be achieved. Vehicle drivers operate in a manner such that the level of risk to which they are exposed is acceptable, and at which they feel comfortable. This level varies, as has been shown earlier, according to sex and age, and must also vary from one individual to another. However, in any given population of drivers, there must be an average level of acceptable risk, and this will be constant or change slowly with time. This being so, the effect of increasing collective skill must be a reduction in the rate at which accidents occur, and hence a reduction in the fatality rate.

The argument set out above is concerned with the way in which human behaviour affects safety. But surely, it might be said, technology must have some influence. What about four-wheel brakes, airbags, crashworthiness, etc.?

There is, indeed, no doubt about the positive contribution that technology has made to road safety. During the period reviewed here, the handleability, reliability and mechanical strength of vehicles – particularly motorcars – have improved enormously, as, to a lesser extent, have the roads on which they run. However, technology does not sit behind the steering wheel of a motorcar. This seat is occupied by a human being, and it is the human population of drivers that is the final arbiter of road safety.

There must, however, be a relationship between these two factors. Thus, it would seem reasonable to suppose that the advance of science and its applications make it possible to improve safety and reduce road casualties, but that human behaviour determines whether or not this should happen, and if so, at what pace. The record for roads in Great Britain, enumerated here, provides a good example of this relationship. Technical improvements to vehicles have been continuous ever since the internal combustion engine was invented. But, with road safety this was not the case: before 1934 fatality rates increased; subsequently they fell.

It is proposed, therefore, that technical development should be regarded as an essential, but permissive, factor in the improvement of safety, but that the pace at which fatality rates fall is determined by the human population concerned.

1.15 Summary and conclusion

Thus, fatal accidents are not random events, having no connection with one another. Their incidence correlates inversely with economic growth such that, as a rule, the more prosperous nations have a lower accident mortality.

Detailed examination of fatal road accidents in Britain shows that fatalities occur in a highly ordered fashion with respect to time. The annual proportional fall in the fatality rate is a constant or slowly varying quantity, such that the change of the casualty rate with time can be represented by a simple exponential trend curve. Also, the proportional spread of data relative to the trend curve is constant. The ordered reduction in road accident fatality rate began spontaneously in 1935, after a period during which the fatality rate increased. These features may only be discerned by analysing the historical record of road accident deaths; they were not ordained by any authority, nor would it be possible for that to happen.

Taking these facts together with the physical character of road transport, it is concluded that the regulated fall of fatality rates results from a subconscious development of skill on the part of the population of road users and, in particular, of vehicle drivers. It is suggested that technological change has an indirect influence: technical developments make an improvement in safety possible, but the population of vehicle drivers will determine the rate of fall of road deaths, and whether or not this will occur.

These conclusions have very profound implications. It is commonly accepted, at least in developed countries, that safety can be assured by devising laws, regulations and procedures based on conscious, rational thought. It would appear, however, that in the case of road transport, fatality rates are regulated and reduced at a satisfactory rate by a non-conscious and non-rational process, and that it is the population of road users, not their supposed rulers, that is responsible for this benefit.

Would it then be politic to scrap road safety laws and regulations, on the grounds that they have had no discernable effect on the historical record, other than, perhaps, an unfavourable one?

It will be evident that a similar dilemma will present itself when considering other human activities, so it will be appropriate to revert to such questions in the final chapter of this book. In the meantime, there is much further evidence to consider.

2
Fatality and loss rates in transport and industry

In this chapter it is proposed to examine and analyse the historical records for air, land and sea transport, for British manufacturing industry, and those for oil and gas exploration, production, and processing. But, before embarking on the task, it will be useful to consider some general topics.

2.1 The theory of accidents

In Chapter 1 it was asserted that there is no generally accepted theory of accidents. Whilst this is quite correct, there exists nevertheless a general opinion that all accidents have a *cause*, that it is the duty of safety experts to identify such causes, and that safety can best be assured by their elimination. Thus, if accident mortality amongst young male civilians increased during wartime, this must have been due to the black-out, not to a change in human behaviour. The cause-and-effect theory treats the human population, or the individuals of whom it is composed, as passive objects whose behaviour is determined by external circumstances. According to the human factor theory, on the other hand, the population acts collectively in a purposeful way, such that fatality rates increase or decrease in a controlled manner and, if external circumstances have any effect, it is to cause year-to-year fluctuations. The human factor theory is, of course, the one which is adopted by this book.

In Chapter 1 it was found that the plot of road accident fatality rates against time showed an abrupt transformation from an upward to a downward trend. This transformation took place in a relatively short time, certainly in less than 1 year. Now the material factors that may be considered to improve road safety include such items as better steering and brakes, improved roads and road markings and more lighting. All such developments, however, take place over periods of several years, and cannot possibly account for a sudden change. Several of the records that are considered in this chapter show similar abrupt changes. It was suggested in Chapter 1 that, in the case of fatal road accidents in Great Britain, the change to a downward trend in fatality rates was due to a change in attitudes on the part of drivers, and that this change was brought about by public concern about the rising number of road deaths. Other, similar changes also occur following a period of increasing fatality rates or losses. It is not surprising that looming disaster should have a sobering effect.

Thus, the cause-and-effect theory is not consistent with the historic records of accidents. It is not suggested, of course, that causes of accidents do not exist. An aircraft pilot attempting a visual approach to a remote airfield in Afghanistan is clearly at greater risk than one making an instrument-aided landing at Chicago Airport. Rather, it is proposed that the human population is collectively responsible for the trend of fatality rate (whether this should be increasing or decreasing with time, and at what rate) but that individual accidents are influenced by local conditions. Thus, the degree of scatter of data will be affected by the variability of local circumstances.

Nor is it suggested that accidents should not be investigated. It is normal engineering practice to make such investigations with a view to establishing causes, and to determine whether or not there were any defects in design, construction, inspection or maintenance that might need amendment. In the present scheme of things, such activities fall into the same category as technical improvements: they contribute to the possibility of safer operations. But the human population has the final say.

2.2 Safety criteria

It is implied by the model that was set up in Chapter 1 (and indeed, by common sense) that fatal accidents result from an error of judgement on the part of the individual, and that fatality rates fall when such errors occur at a lower rate. There is not, however, a one-to-one relationship between these two quantities. In airline operations, for example, a single error may result in a large number of deaths. As a rule, and in the case of road transport, the fatality rate is a sound criterion but, for aircraft and also for shipping, the proportional annual loss is a better measure. In the case of ocean-going ships, loss of life has only recently been recorded, so here there is no choice. Railways present a special problem, which will be discussed in the appropriate section.

2.3 Analysing the historical data

Details of tools, methods and the mathematical background are given in Chapter 5. Essential steps are firstly, to make a plot of the relevant data against time, then to decide to which periods particular trends apply, and finally to analyse these periods separately.

In the case of an exponential fall in fatality or loss rates (in this book designated the 'normal' case) the plot has two basic parameters: the proportional gradient and the proportional standard deviation, as noted in Chapter 1.

The proportional gradient of an exponential curve is equal to the gradient at any point on the curve divided by the value shown by the curve at the same point. Thus, when the trend curve represents a plot of fatality or loss rates R as a function of time t,

$$\frac{1}{R}\frac{\mathrm{d}R}{\mathrm{d}t} = b \qquad [2.1]$$

where b is a constant. Suppose the value of b is –0.05, this means that the value of R according to the trend curve falls by 5% each year (the unit of time having earlier been set at 1 year).

Data points scatter on either side of the trend curve, forming a scatter band. It is found empirically that the width of the scatter band, measured vertically, is proportional to the corresponding value of R predicted by the trend curve. Thus, it is possible to establish a constant average proportional half-width for the scatter band, which is the relative standard deviation σ_r. Provided that the frequency distribution of data conforms to a normal pattern, then about 95% of the points should fall between the boundaries set by a distance of $2\sigma_r R$ on either side of the trend curve. Where appropriate, such boundaries will be shown on the plots for transport and industry.

Much prominence has been given here to the exponentially represented trend, and it has indeed been the most common type during the twentieth century. There are, however, cases where a straight line gives a better representation (usually where the rate increases with time) and occasionally the plot takes a sinusoidal form.

2.4 Fatality and loss rates in transport and industry

Those instances where there is an exponential fall of the loss rate will be considered first.

2.4.1 Air passenger transport

The record to be considered here is that supplied by the Boeing Company of Seattle, USA. This covers commercial passenger jet aircraft operating domestically and internationally. The record starts in 1964, a few years after the introduction of jet aircraft on the transatlantic route. An annual report is published, giving details of aircraft numbers, losses and fatalities. It also includes an analysis of the causes of accidents to aircraft. These are divided into 'air crew' (i.e. human error) and mechanical failure. The predominant cause is 'air crew'. The journal *Flight International* also publishes annually a listing of the previous year's aircraft crashes, and here, too, the predominant cause of accidents is pilot error. Bearing in mind that mechanical failure represents human error at one stage removed, these results are consistent with the conclusions of Chapter 1 of this book.

It was suggested earlier that, where a singular error could result in large numbers of deaths, the proportional loss of units would be a better measure of safety than the fatality rate. Accordingly, Fig. 2.1 plots the annual percentage of jet aircraft suffering a total loss between 1964 and 2000. The annual proportional decline of the loss rate is high, being 5.5%.

There are, of course, a number of factors that would favour this state of affairs. The system is particularly amenable to technological development such as automatic controls, instrument landing systems and others. Aircrew are carefully selected and trained. And, there is a commercial incentive: jet aircraft are exceedingly costly. These are speculative considerations, of course, in the end; improvements of the loss rate are due to the aircrews themselves.

The relative standard deviation is also high, being equal to 0.29. Lines corresponding to the trend curve value times $(1 + 2\sigma)$ and $(1 - 2\sigma)$, respectively, are plotted on the figure (the lower line is almost horizontal). It may be recalled that such lines should form a boundary to the scatter band of data points, and should enclose about 95% of these points. Such is indeed the case here.

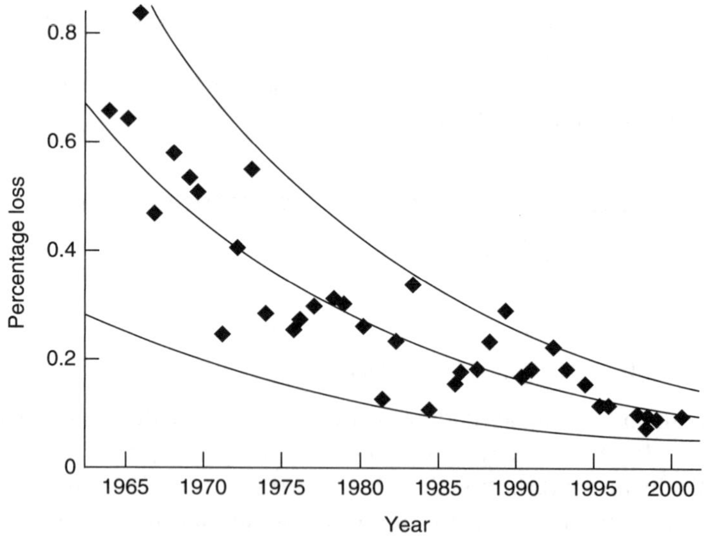

2.1 Percentage of the world's fleet of commercial jet aircraft suffering a complete loss 1964–2000. Annual fall of loss rate: 5.5%. Relative standard deviation: 0.29.

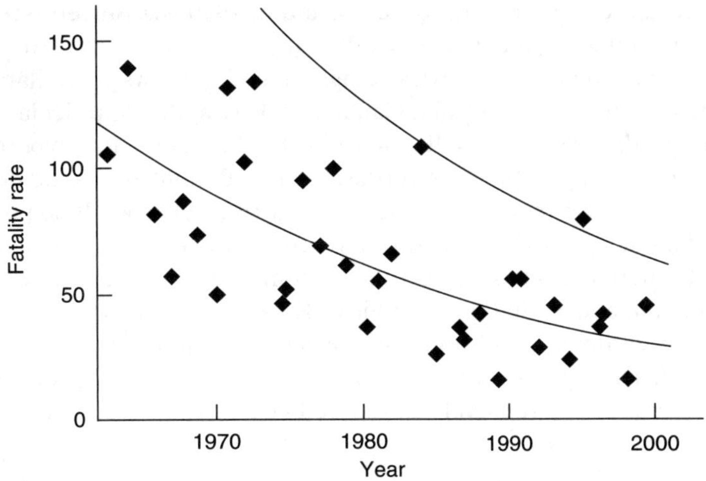

2.2 Fatality rate per million departures due to accidents to passenger jet aircraft world-wide 1964–2000. Annual fall of fatality rate: 3.5%. Relative standard deviation: 0.48. The fatality rate for 1966, not shown, was 287. The lower scatter boundary lies too close to the x axis to be shown.

An alternative measure of safety, which has been used in the case of railway accidents, is the number of deaths per million departures, or take-offs. Figure 2.2 plots the relevant data for jet aircraft from 1964 to 2000. The rate declines at 3.5% annually, which is quite satisfactory but, as would be expected, there is a wide scatter band.

Because the number of deaths per accident is high, these figures do not provide a good estimate of the risk to an individual, which is better measured by the annual proportional loss divided by the annual number of departures. According to this measure, the risk of death due to a major air accident would have been, for a traveller taking one flight in a year, one in one hundred million in 1964 and 5 in a hundred billion in 2000. Few airline passengers would believe such estimates: indeed, they are so small as to be meaningless. The best that can be said is that large aircraft provide a relatively safe mode of travel.

2.4.2 Road transport

International comparisons

Figure 1.2 of Chapter 1 shows the inverse relationship that exists at any given time between fatality rates due to road accidents and national prosperity, as measured by the per capita gross domestic product, or national output per head. The number of motor vehicles per head of population is also a measure of national prosperity, and in 1970 R.J. Smeed (see Appendix) showed that a similar reciprocal relationship exists between this quantity and road death rates. Accordingly, Fig. 2.3 shows a similar plot for European countries, Australia, Canada and New Zealand, Iceland, Japan, Korea and the USA. The solid curve in the diagram is the hyperbola that best fits the data points, which represent annual number of road deaths per 10000 vehicles against the number of motor vehicles per 1000 population. Figure 2.3 suggests that the safest place to travel in by road would be Iceland, where the fatality rate is 0.4, as compared with 1.5 in Great Britain, 5.8 in Poland and 8.0 in the Republic of Korea. All these risks are, of course, modest as compared with those countries at the left-hand end of the plot in Fig. 1.2. The significance of the new plot is that the reciprocal relationship also applies to relatively developed countries at the beginning of the twenty-first century.

Number of road deaths

It was shown in Chapter 1 that the fatality rate due to road accidents in Great Britain (and, by implication, in other developed countries) varies in a regulated manner. It was proposed that the fall in the fatality rate resulted from a development of human skill, and that the pace with which fatality rates declined was determined by the rate of development of skill. Thus,

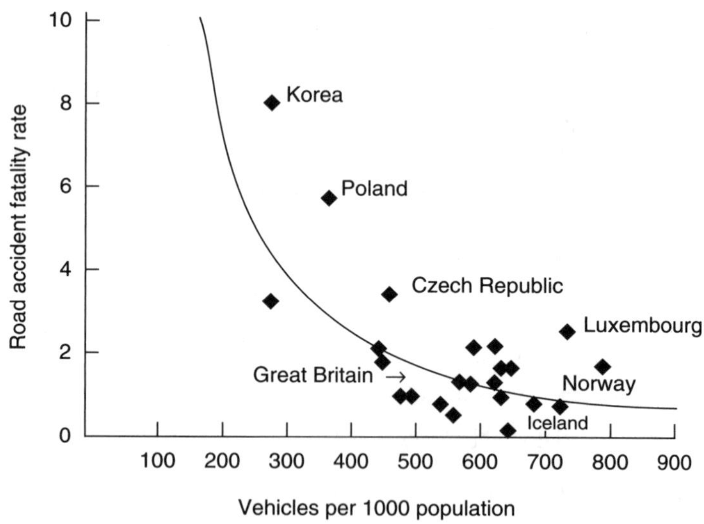

2.3 Annual fatality rate per 10000 vehicles due to road accidents as a function of the number of motor vehicles per head of population for various countries of Europe plus Australia, Canada, New Zealand, Iceland, Japan, Korea and the USA.

for any given year, the number of road deaths will be equal to the fatality rate per vehicle multiplied by the number of vehicles on the road.

In Great Britain, vehicle numbers increased steadily but rather slowly until 1939. During the war they fell to a low point in 1943. Then from 1944 to 2000 (and beyond) they increased in a linear manner, but much more rapidly than during the pre-war period. Figure 2.4 illustrates these trends for the period 1926–1955. There are two features of special interest about this plot. Firstly, the transformation from an upward to a downward trend in fatality rates which occurred in 1934 is not reflected at all in vehicle numbers. Thus, fatality rates and vehicle numbers vary independently. Secondly, the upturn in numbers started in 1944, before the end of the war and before any motorcars had been manufactured for civilian use. There were, no doubt, many pre-war vehicles stowed away in garages, awaiting better times. And, evidently, by 1944 owners had decided that things were indeed on the mend.

From 1944 onwards, the number of registered vehicles (most of which were motorcars) increased in a steady, linear fashion. Figure 2.5 shows the plot for 1980–2000, which is typical of the period. The trend 'curve' is a straight line, with a constant annual numerical increase (in contrast with exponential growth, where there is a constant *proportional* increase). Data points form a continuous chain, which snakes up and down inside the scatter boundaries: plots of human population growth for the same period

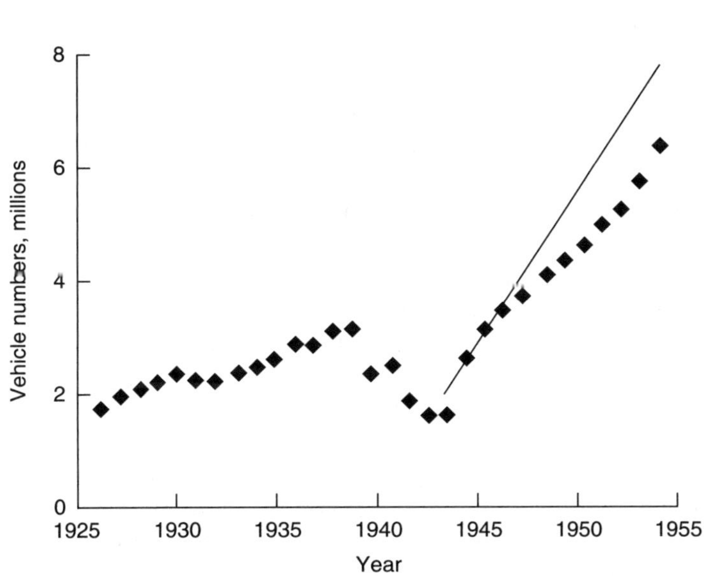

2.4 Number (millions) of motor vehicles registered in Great Britain 1926–1955. The solid line is part of the trend line for 1944–2000.

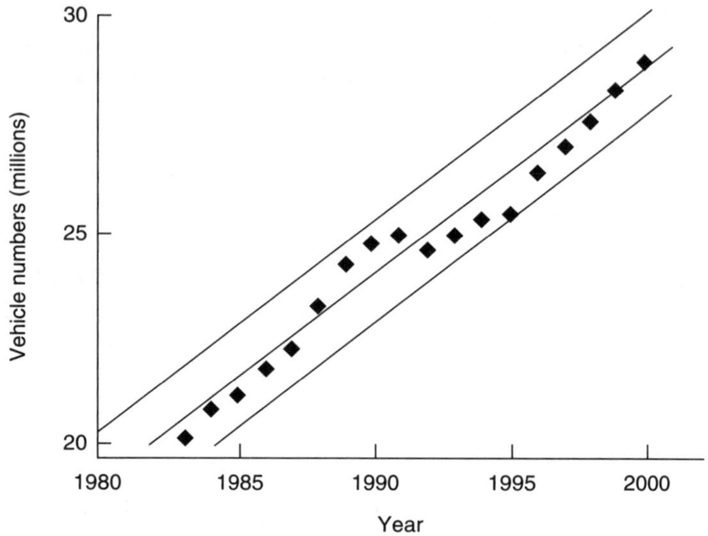

2.5 Number of motor vehicles registered in Great Britain from 1945–2000, showing detail for the period 1980–2000. Average annual increase: 0.48 millions. Relative standard deviation: 0.038.

are very similar to that shown in Fig. 2.5. There is indeed a relationship between human and motor vehicle growth. The trend line may be represented by the equation

$$n = ct + d \qquad [2.2]$$

where t is time and c and d are constants.

Most of the historical records examined previously in this book have been concerned with accident mortality or fatality rates and, in most instances, the plot of such data shows an exponential fall. Figure 2.6 illustrates an exceptional case: that of annual road death numbers in Great Britain between 1926 and 1934. This indicates a rising linear trend, which differs from Fig. 2.5 in that data points in Fig. 2.6 are scattered in a random fashion. In the case of vehicle numbers, the data points are connected one with another. Random scatter is characteristic of fatal accident data, and appears also in plots where there is an exponential fall.

There is good reason for this observed difference. There are two essential requirements for an increase in vehicle numbers. Firstly, the material well-being of the country must improve, such that a higher proportion of the population can afford a motorcar. Secondly, there must be developments in manufacture and infrastructure; increased vehicle production, fuel distribution, better roads and so forth. These are physical changes that can only be accomplished progressively; hence the progressive nature of the data plot.

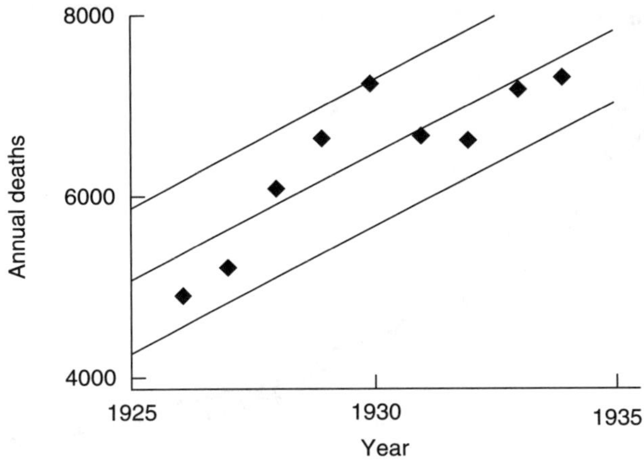

2.6 Number of persons killed annually on roads in Great Britain 1926–1934. Annual increase: 419. Relative standard deviation: 0.065.

The incidence of fatal accidents, however, is not constrained in this way. Whilst a general trend is established in the manner described earlier, there is no physical link that would connect the results for successive years.

A similar argument applies in the case of other modes of transport and for industry.

The other feature that is desirable to note here is that, in the case of an exponential fall in mortality or fatality rates, the width of the scatter band falls proportionally with the trend curve value of the rate. Figure 2.7 illustrates this characteristic: it is a plot of British road accident fatality rates from 1945 to 2000. The scatter band of linear plots, such as those in Figs. 2.5 and 2.6, are, on the other hand, constant in width. Thus the equation for the two scatter boundaries for the straight-line plot is:

$$R = ct + d \pm 2\sigma \qquad [2.3]$$

whilst that for the exponential case is

$$R = (1 \pm 2\sigma_r)(ae^{bt}) \qquad [2.4]$$

where σ is the standard deviation and σ_r is the relative or proportional standard deviation. These relationships are set out in formal detail in Chapter 5.

Relative standard deviations are non-dimensional and are comparable, regardless of the activity they represent.

To return to matters of more immediate interest: it has been established that, for the period of 1945 to 2000, fatality rates in accidents on British roads fell exponentially, whilst the numbers of vehicles increased in a linear

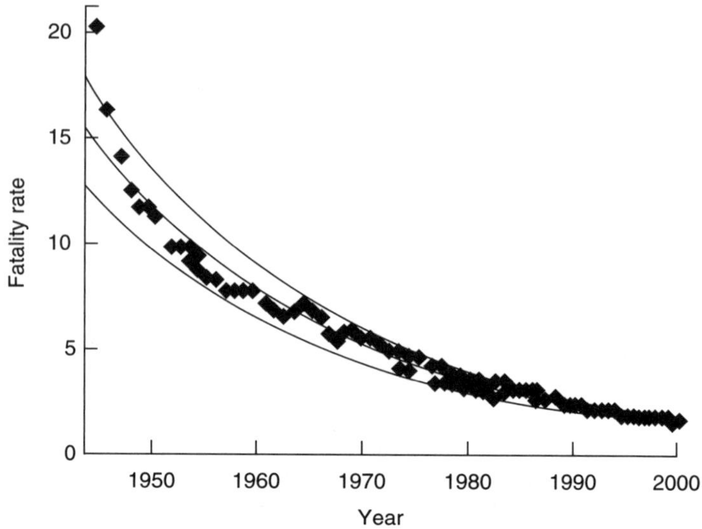

2.7 Fatality rate per 10000 vehicles on roads in Great Britain 1945–2000, showing how width of scatter band diminishes in proportion to the fatality rate. Relative standard deviation: 0.089.

manner. It is therefore possible to obtain a trend curve for the number of road deaths by multiplying the two relevant equations:

$$n = (ct + d)(ae^{bt}) \tag{2.5}$$

In Fig. 2.8 this expression is plotted together with the relevant data points. The trend curve rises to a peak in 1962 and eventually takes a more or less exponential form. Early data points were distorted downwards by the shortage of motorcars following the Second World War; otherwise there is a good agreement.

The maximum of Equation 2.5 occurs where:

$$t = \frac{-1}{b}\left(\frac{1 + bd}{e}\right) \tag{2.6}$$

that is, in 1962. The maximum according to the data plot was in 1966. Prior to this date, the rising number of vehicles was dominant in determining the annual number of road deaths; subsequently, the exponential fall in fatality rate became the more important factor.

2.4.3 Shipping

For reasons that were stated earlier, the criterion of safety used here is the annual percentage loss of ships. Ship losses may be measured in numbers

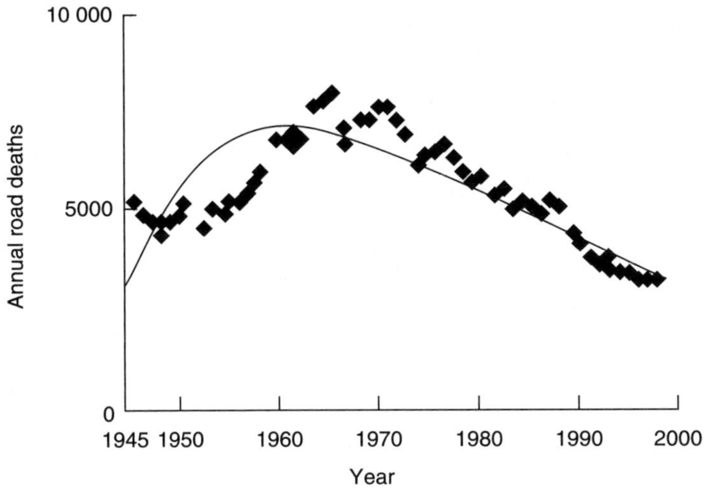

2.8 Numbers of persons killed annually on roads in Great Britain 1945–2000, with trend curve.

or tonnage, but numbers are judged to be more appropriate. Data are from Lloyd's Register of Shipping, London, and are for steamships and motor ships with a displacement of 100 tons or more. The coverage is for commercial ocean-going ships world-wide; the period is from 1900 to 2000. Sailing ships operated commercially up to the 1930s; these have been excluded because of their intrinsically higher rate of loss.

Figures for human loss have only been recorded and published during recent years and the record is not long enough to justify analysis. However, the proportional loss of ships provides a rough estimate of the proportional loss of crews.

Figure 2.9 is the relevant plot. It shows a characteristic exponential fall. Data for the two war periods, when losses were very high, have been excluded.

The number of vessels in the world's commercial steam and motor ships fleet began to rise sharply after 1965, corresponding with a growth in world trade. Loss rates started to increase at almost the same time, and continued to do so for several years. This tendency is, in a sense, opposite to that observed earlier, where, over a long term, fatality rates were found to correlate with an increase in prosperity. This tendency for increased recklessness during an economic boom is not uncommon, and will be considered in Chapter 4.

2.4.4 British manufacturing industry

The term 'manufacturing' is used here to denote productive work that is carried out in factories. Factory work began in England in the middle of

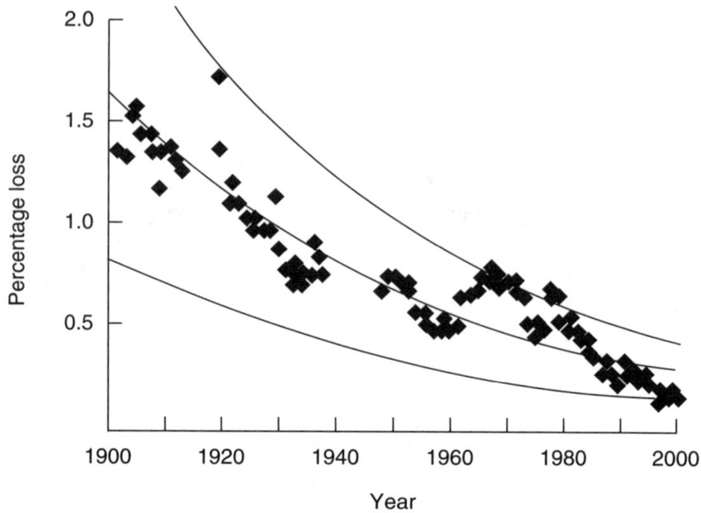

2.9 Percentage loss of merchant ocean-going ships from the world's fleet 1900–2000. Data for the periods of the two World Wars, where available, have been omitted. Annual fall of loss rate: 1.78%. Relative standard deviation: 0.25.

the eighteenth century for the production of cloth. Factories provided a means of transmitting power to machines, which could produce goods more cheaply and of better quality; the power source was originally water, then during the nineteenth century, steam, and later electricity. In the early days, factory conditions were far from ideal and, during the nineteenth century, the British parliament passed a series of factory acts, initially to control the use of child labour, then to promote safe working methods. At a relatively late stage, the reporting of fatal accidents was required, such that records are available from 1880 onwards.

The plot for the manufacturing industry divides into three phases. The first of these is shown in Fig. 2.10a. This comprises data for the period 1880–1895. The trend is downwards; the trend curve indicates a diminution of the fatality rate of slightly less than 1% annually. There would be some question as to the significance of such a modest fall except that, during the following period, 1896–1920 (shown in Fig. 2.10b) there was a relatively rapid rise. This was not a statistical quirk; annual deaths from factory accidents rose from 487 in 1896 to 1175 in 1920.

There was then a sharp drop in annual deaths from 1178 to 751 in 1921. This initiated a period of exponential fall, which is illustrated in Fig. 2.11. There is no doubt about the significance of this second decline, which was at a rate of 3.2% annually, and which has been maintained over a long period of time.

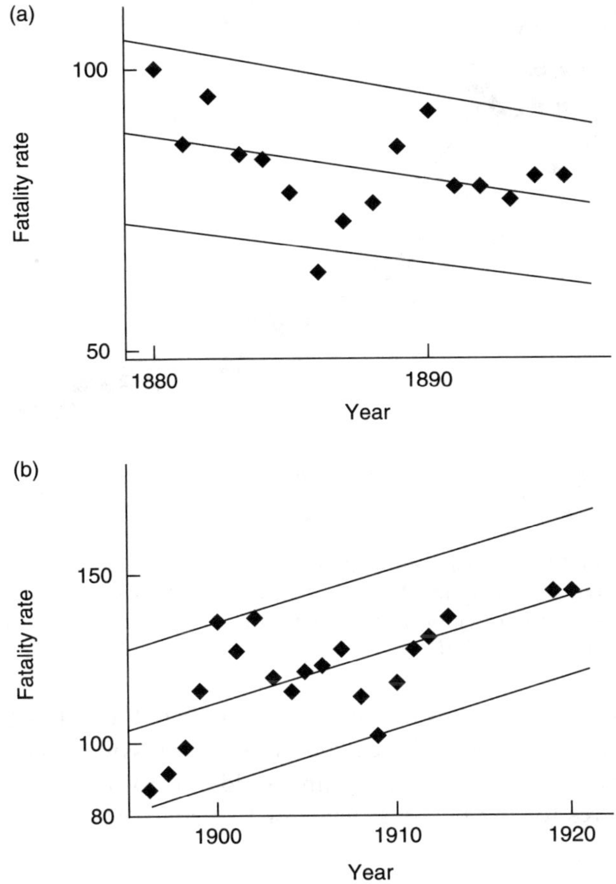

2.10 Annual fatality rate per million employees in British factories (a) 1880–1895 (b) 1896–1920. The relative standard deviations: (a) 0.09 (b) 0.11.

2.5 Comment

It may be recalled that, by 1880, accident mortality – that is, fatality rates from all types of accident – was falling in Britain. This further reinforces the view that the fall shown in Fig. 2.10a was a real trend. Furthermore, it will be seen that the width of the scatter band is proportional to the fatality rate predicted by the trend curve, as with other exponential falls.

Thus, in the main, fatality rates in British factories conform to the general pattern. The rising trend between 1896 and 1920, however, is anomalous and difficult to explain. The number of accidental deaths rose to a peak in 1918, was maintained at a high level in 1919 and 1920, then fell sharply in

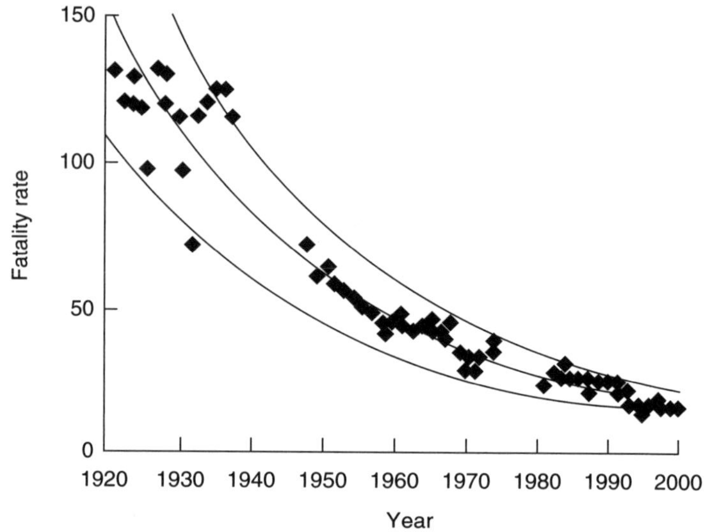

2.11 Annual fatality rate per million employees due to accidents in British manufacturing industry from 1920 to 2000. Annual fall: 3.2%, relative standard deviation: 0.15. Data for the two World War periods have not been included.

1921. There was a period of naval re-armament prior to the 1914–1918 war, and it is conceivable that patriotic zeal amongst factory workers could have resulted in an increased accident rate. This would not, however, explain the high fatality figures for the post-war years of 1919 and 1920.

2.6 Exceptions to the normal pattern

The activities described so far in this chapter conform to a normal pattern; that is, for all or most of the recorded period, the fatality rate diminishes exponentially. The following sections detail those instances which, in one way or another, deviate from this norm.

2.6.1 Motorcycling in Britain

It will be generally conceded that a motorcycle is intrinsically less safe than a four-wheeled vehicle. Motorcycle riders are exposed to the weather; the vehicle is less stable; and in the event of a collision, its occupants are likely to be thrown on to the road, possibly in front of oncoming traffic. Such prior reasoning would suggest that motorcyclists should suffer a substantially higher rate of fatal accidents than the average for all road users.

In fact, this was not the case during the earlier years of the twentieth century. Figure 2.12a compares the fatality rate per 10000 motorcycles with

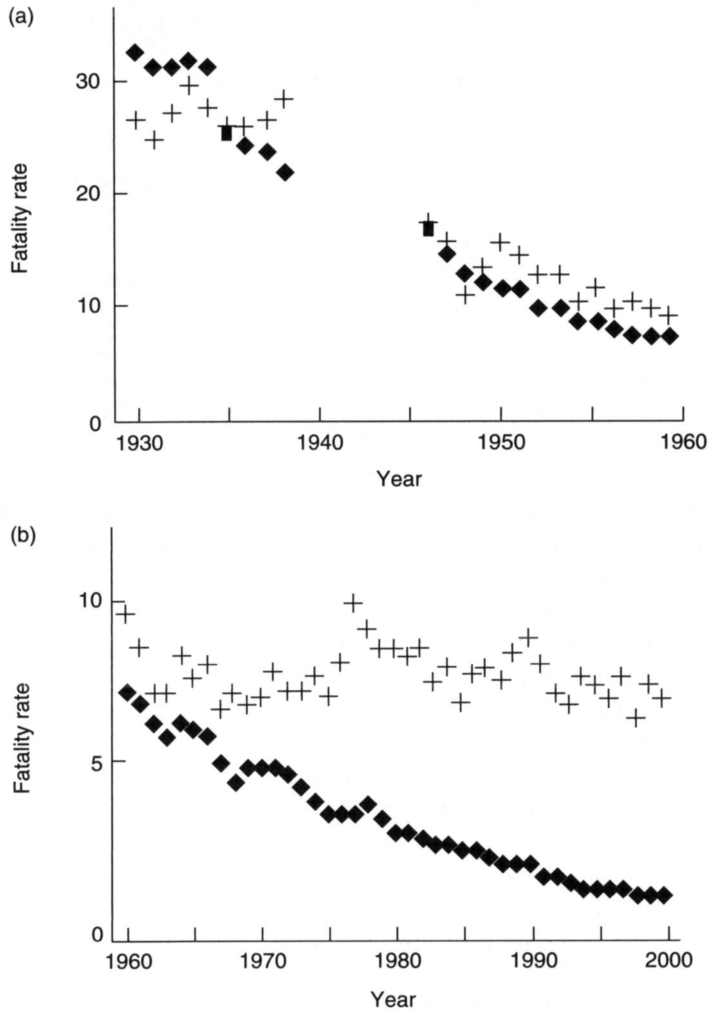

2.12 Annual fatality rate due to accidents on British roads per 10 000 vehicles, comparing those for motorcycle riders (+) with data for all road users ◆ (a) 1930–1959 (b) 1960–2000.

that for all road users during the period 1930–1959, but omits data for the war years. Prior to 1960, the plot for motorcycle fatalities follows the general trend almost exactly. Before the war, it was linear with a slight upward tendency; afterwards, it followed a similar downward exponential course, just marginally higher than the data for all users, which was, of course, primarily that for the motorcar.

Indeed, the motorcycle was, during this period, the poor man's motorcar. With a sidecar attached, it was possible to take the whole family for a spin on a Sunday in summer. Family or no, the motorcyclist of that time was able to match his skills and behaviour almost exactly to that of the motorist.

Then, in the early 1960s, the situation changed. The process described in Chapter 1 whereby motoring ceased to be a sport and became part of daily routine, with a corresponding fall in fatality rates, operated in reverse: motorcycling ceased to emulate the motorcar and became a sport. This sport, moreover, was consistent with the spirit of the time, dominated by young men. Figure 2.12b shows motorcycling fatality rates from 1960 to 2000. The rate has stopped declining and fluctuates about a more-or-less constant level. The result has been a significant number of premature deaths, mostly of young men.

The changes recorded above must have been influenced by technological and economic development. Early motorcars were exceedingly expensive, and were only affordable by a small number of rich people. However, a general rise of income level combined with a fall in manufacture cost soon led to mass ownership. This change from a generally leisured to a working section of the population would undoubtedly have favoured the transition from a rising to a falling fatality rate. Then, a further increase in prosperity made it possible for young men to acquire motorcycles and create a new, hazardous sport.

These points of special interest arise from this particular record. Firstly, despite the greater risks pertaining to their machines, motorcyclists were able, during the 1930–1959 period, to operate at a safety level similar to that of four-wheeled vehicles. Secondly, the transformation from caution to a controlled level of recklessness was quite indubitably the result of a change in attitude; no material circumstance could possibly have given rise to such a change.

Thirdly, the record for the post-1960 period poses several problems. The trend is linear and almost level, and this condition is self-evidently controlled. British motorcyclists are not all young men: a significant proportion are middle-aged. It is possible, therefore, that a young minority is responsible for the fatality rate. If so, the means of control could be similar to that proposed in Chapter 1, except that, instead of being comfortable with declining risk, the minority is concerned to maintain a level of risk higher than that to which the common road user is exposed.

Regardless of the truth or otherwise of such speculations, the post-1960 record for motorcyclists is clear evidence of the human control of accident fatality rates. It is also characterised by a curious spikiness, both before and after 1960. The human control does not, in this case, operate smoothly.

2.6.2 British railways

Passenger railways started in 1830 with the opening of the Liverpool to Manchester line. In Britain, their expansion, as measured by the number of passenger journeys, was continuous until 1920 after which their use (again measured as passenger journeys) remained more or less steady until the last few years of the twentieth century, when there was a modest increase.

Passenger safety has always been a prior concern, and in 1871 legislation was passed, requiring that details of railway accidents be reported. So, data on passenger fatalities are available from 1875 onwards. The option of measuring safety by the annual proportion of vehicles lost is not practicable in the case of railways, and the criterion used here is the annual number of passengers killed in train accidents per billion passenger journeys. The advantage of this measure is that it makes possible a comparison with other forms of transport; the comparison shows that railways provide one of the safest forms of transport. The disadvantage, which was discussed earlier under the heading 'Safety Criteria', is that of extreme variability. Most railway accidents result in a small number of casualties but, from time to time, large numbers of people are killed. Such accidents receive wide publicity and cause much public concern.

There are other complications, and, in particular, the trend of data between 1875 and 2000 is not uniform. Between 1875 and 1920, the fatality rate fell exponentially in the normal manner. Then, from 1921 to 1952 the fatality rate increased. In 1952 there was a double collision at Harrow and Wealdstone in which more than 100 people were killed. Subsequently, the rate fell sharply and in the final phase, between 1953 and 2000, there was a gradual fall.

Figure 2.13 is the relevant plot. Earliest data are available as 10-year averages. This eliminates the year-to-year variations, and the plot for the first period is quite smooth. After 1920, data are plotted annually, and the result is not so smooth. The trend lines shown for 1921–1952 and 1953–2000 are a least-squares fit (see Chapter 5) to these annual figures.

In the sector concerned with British manufacturing industry, 1920 was found to be a year of change, but in the opposite sense: from a relatively reckless period to one in which fatality rates fell in a more-or-less ordered fashion.

In Fig. 2.13 the exponentially falling trend curve for the first period has been extended to the year 2000, and it will be seen that the upwardly deviant trend lines eventually fall close to this extrapolation. It is a pattern similar to that observed for fatality rates in wartime, and it has been suggested that the upward deviation was due to a small minority (probably young men), that the major part of the population remained on its original

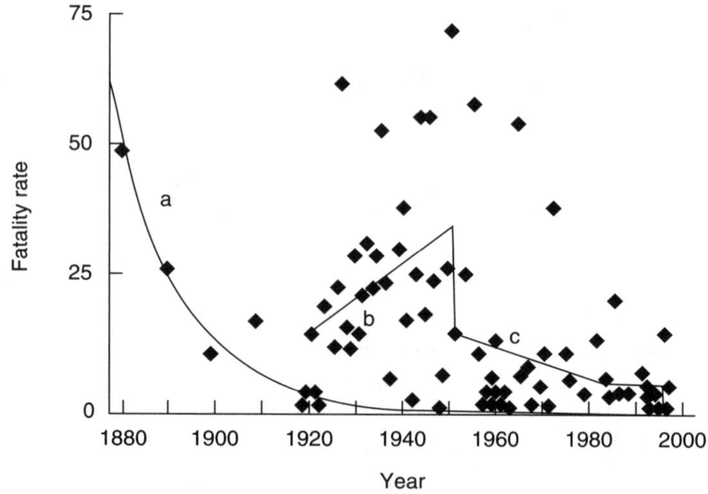

2.13 Annual fatality rate per billion journeys for passengers on British railways during successive periods 1875–2000 (a) 1875–1930 (b) 1921–1952 (c) 1953–2000.

track, and at the end of the war the errant minority returned to normal behaviour. A similar model could apply to the railways, except that the return to normality was precipitated not by the end of the war, but by the shock of the Harrow and Wealdstone accident.

As for the rising trend after 1920; this paralleled a period of unrest and disaffection that was associated with the economic depression after the 1914–1918 war and which was manifest in the general strike of 1926.

2.6.3 The oil industry

Hydrocarbon production falls into three phases: exploration and production, processing and marketing. The first step is to locate viable reservoirs of oil and gas, and to then drill wells and extract as much as possible. Secondly, crude oil and untreated gas are processed to obtain marketable products. Thirdly, the products are transported and sold. In this section only the first two phases will be considered.

Offshore oil and gas

Most of the land-based sources of oil, other than those in the Antarctic, have already been located, and in recent years much exploration has been carried out offshore on the continental shelf.

The second half of the twentieth century saw exploration for oil and gas beneath the North Sea, and significant, although rather short-lived, sources were located off the British and Norwegian coasts. Partly as a result of these developments, Det Norske Veritas, a marine inspection organisation located in Oslo, has collected data concerning accidents and fatalities in offshore operations world-wide. The results were published annually between 1964 and 1997, and have subsequently been maintained on a database in Oslo. The document in question, *World Offshore Accident Data* (*WOAD*), is the source for the analysis presented here.

Exploration for oil and gas offshore is carried out using specialised seagoing vessels, whose main purpose is to provide a stable platform from which drilling can take place. The commonest type is the jack-up unit. This is a flat-topped barge to which vertical legs are attached. These legs can be jacked down to the sea bed and then jacked further to raise the barge or platform clear of any impact by waves. If a trial drilling indicates the presence of oil or gas, the well is capped, and the barge is lowered and towed to another promising site. There are several other types of mobile unit: all share the common requirement of maintaining a fixed position and a stable platform. Thus, there are hazards that add on to those normally faced by ships. In addition, the North Sea is a most inhospitable place, where bad weather can produce waves 30 feet in height. Other offshore operations may also face hazardous conditions, and there is good reason to monitor the safety record.

Figure 2.14 is a plot of the percentage loss of mobile offshore units world-wide from 1970 to 1997. This indicates an exponential fall of the loss rate of 6.4% annually: an exceptionally rapid diminution. In 1970 the offshore

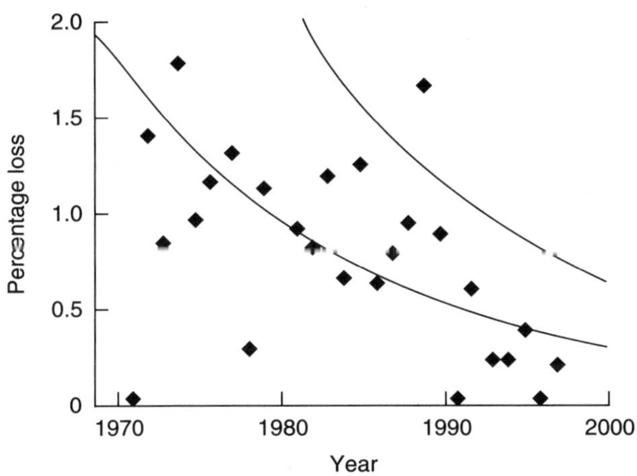

2.14 Percentage loss of mobile craft engaged in oil and gas exploration world-wide 1970–1997. Annual fall of loss rate according to trend curve = 6.4%; zero data points are shown as indicated for 1971. The lower boundary of the scatter band is too close to the x axis to be shown.

mobile loss rate was 2.1%, about three times that of ocean-going ships. By 1997, however, the losses for those two categories were very similar. It is possible that the rate of development of skill operating offshore units has compensated for the inherent problems described above.

The scatter of data is nevertheless very high: the relative standard deviation is 0.65. However, this is not surprising in view of the potential adversities and the high rate of improvement of the loss rate.

A plot of fatality rate against time provides a completely different picture. Figure 2.15 shows annual deaths per 100 units for mobile craft offshore worldwide from 1970 to 1997. This diagram divides into two parts. From 1970 to 1989 there was an intermittent series of years with high and increasing fatality rates, with low values in the intervening years. Overall, there was a steady increasing trend. Then, from 1989 to 1990, a sudden drop occurred, followed by a gradual fall.

The pattern of events is similar to that observed in the case of passenger deaths on British railways (Fig. 2.13). In both industries the sudden drop in fatal accidents occurred after a catastrophe. For the railways, this was a double collision in which over 100 passengers were killed. Offshore, seven vessels were lost in 1989 and, in one of these, 91 men were killed. In both cases a period of reckless behaviour was brought to an end by the shock of a catastrophic accident.

It was suggested that the rise of the railway passenger fatality rate during the early half of the twentieth century was the result of disaffection amongst a minority of railway workers.

This is very unlikely to have been the case with offshore operations. American practice is dominant in oil exploration and production, and

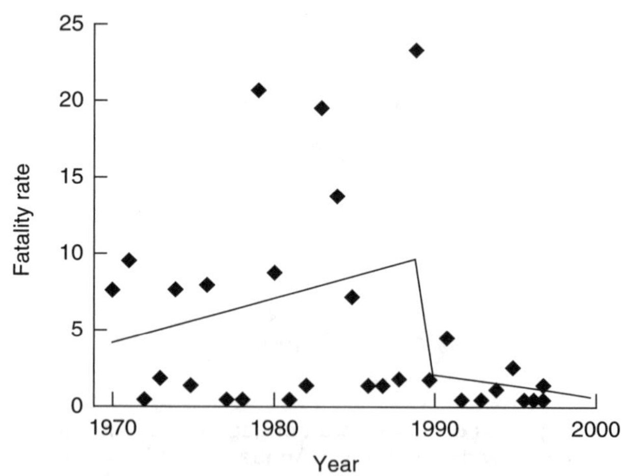

2.15 Annual fatality rate per 100 units for mobile craft operations world-wide 1970–1997.

Americans have a positive attitude to work. Thus, the initially reckless operators were most likely to have resulted from an excess of zeal. Indeed, the greatest loss in 1989 occurred because a mobile unit remained at sea under excessively severe weather conditions.

Fixed offshore units

Once a viable oil or gas field has been located, it is exploited using a fixed unit. There are several types, but the most common is a tubular steel structure that is anchored or tethered to the sea bed, and which supports several platforms or levels, one for drilling, and others for the initial processing of the raw material. In the Mexican Gulf and in the Middle East, units are usually small, but in the North Sea they are generally large. Earlier North Sea structures were none too safe, and the unit operating the Piper Alpha field suffered a severe catastrophic explosion and fire with considerable loss of life. Overall, however, fatality rates are low, and more or less in line with those of shore-based industry.

Hydrocarbon processing

Natural gas, as drawn from the well, consists of a mixture of methane and other gaseous hydrocarbon, together with the vapours of other hydrocarbons that are normally liquid at ambient temperature. A relatively simple process is required to produce methane, which is used domestically for cooking and heating and as a feedstock for petrochemical plant.

Crude oil varies widely in chemical composition and physical properties, but is usually a viscous liquid consisting of a mixture of many hydrocarbons with, as a rule, liquid compounds of sulphur. It is processed in oil refineries, the main products of which are paraffin (kerosene), petrol (gasoline), lubricating oil and heavy fuel oil. Petrochemical plants produce a very wide range of products. Ethylene, a raw material for that ubiquitous plastic, polythene, is one of the more important hydrocarbon products and also one of the most dangerous.

All hydrocarbon processing is, to some degree, hazardous because it deals with volatile, inflammable substances, and because there is always a source of ignition on the plant site. Thus, accidental ruptures can result in devastating fires. Worse still, a failure may release a large cloud of vapour which, when mixed with air, spreads until it reaches a source of heat, is ignited and explodes. Investigators of such explosions rate them in terms of their equivalent in tonnes of TNT, and the resulting cost of repair is counted in tens of millions of dollars.

Marsh and McLennan, insurance brokers and risk consultants of Chicago, USA, maintained and published a record of the 100 largest financial losses due to accidents in the hydrocarbon processing industry world-wide. This is not, of course, a complete tally, but it is quite adequate to indicate trends. It is used here in conjunction with the British Petroleum *Statistical Review of World Energy* to obtain the percentage financial loss due to accidents in oil refineries. In so doing, it is assumed that the price of crude oil is US$100 per tonne. Thus, the percentage loss for any given year is the annual financial loss due to accidents divided by the annual production of crude oil in tonnes. The results of such calculations for 1975–2001 are plotted in Fig. 2.16.

For the period 1975–1993, this plot is remarkably similar to that in Fig. 2.15. A series of data points indicating a low and almost steady level of accidental loss is interspersed with increasingly high yearly losses. These culminate in a peak in 1992, when the total loss was US$558.7 million. Then there was an abrupt fall to US$72.4 million in 1993. Subsequently, there appears to have been a resumption of the upward trend, but this remains to be confirmed.

Figures 2.15 and 2.16 represent two very different types of activity but they share a common feature: in both cases, American technology and practice are predominant. Thus, in both instances, there is a high degree of uniformity in spite of the international distribution of operations and, although oil exploration and oil refining are very different types of activity, it is equally possible to operate an offshore mobile craft or an oil refinery either recklessly or cautiously.

The present author became aware of the data collected by Marsh and McLennan prior to 1992. At the time, annual losses were mounting steadily,

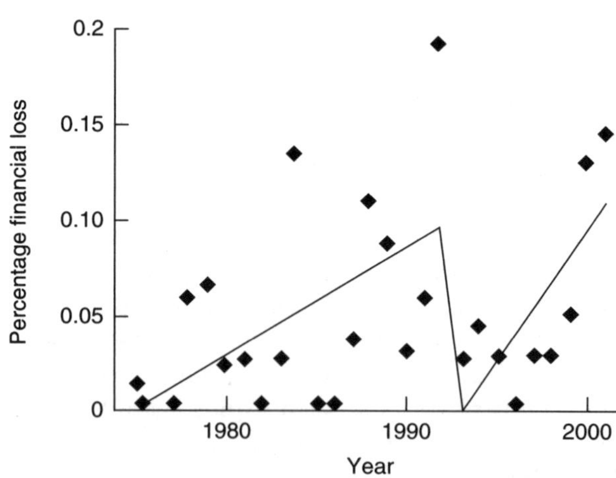

2.16 Annual percentage financial loss due to catastrophic accidents in petroleum refineries world-wide 1975–2001.

which was at odds with the records of other industries which showed a decline in loss rates. Moreover, those concerned with safety in the oil industry were very well aware of its hazards, and defensive procedures had been set up by government agencies and by the industry itself. At the time, I was a devotee of the cause-and-effect theory of accidents, and spent some time looking for material circumstances – increased concentration of assets on the refinery plant, higher incidence of vapour cloud explosions and so on – that could be used to explain the phenomenon. Then came a later edition of the Marsh and McLennan report, which showed the dramatic fall between 1992 and 1993. It was immediately apparent that this fall could not possibly be the result of any physical change: the time scale was too short and anyway no observable change had occurred. Therefore, it was evidently a human cause: that the plant operators were equally responsible for the rising trends of losses and for their sudden fall. Then if, in such a safety-regulated industry, the working population itself regulated the loss rate and hence the level of safety, this must be the case generally.

The late 1980s and early 1990s were periods of some disturbance in the economies of some developed nations. In Britain there was a stock market collapse in 1987, a housing market collapse in 1988, and a fall in national output in 1990. It is not impossible that the same prevalent mood could have shaped the records of offshore fatalities and financial loss in oil refining. In both cases this plot showed a steady rise followed by a sudden fall: very similar to that of a stock market collapse. In all of these instances, it may be supposed that the initial reckless period is fuelled by a mood of excessive optimism: eventually the bubble of optimism bursts, and there is a collapse.

2.7 Summary and comment

This chapter starts by considering some general topics. In particular, it is noted that, although there is no generally agreed theory of accidents, there exists a widely accepted view that accidents are the result of material circumstances: that every accident has a *cause* and, by implication, the incidence of fatal accidents can be reduced by discovering such causes and eliminating them. For convenience, this view is known here as the cause-and-effect theory.

By contrast, it is proposed in Chapter 1 of this book that accidents result from human error, and that the development of collective skill by national populations reduces the incidence of such errors, such that fatal accident and loss rates are reduced in a controlled and regulated manner.

It is noted that, in the case of aircraft, railways and ships, a single error may result in large numbers of casualties, and that the loss rate may be a better measure of safety than the fatality rate.

Fatality and loss rates for the various modes of transport and for some productive activities are detailed and analysed in the light of the model proposed in Chapter 1. Accordingly, topics are divided into 'normal': that is where, in the main, fatality or loss rates fall exponentially with time, and exceptions, where, to a significant extent, this is not the case.

Road transport in general, aircraft and shipping, and the British manufacturing industry fall into the normal category. Motorcycling and rail transport in Britain, and exploration and hydrocarbon processing in the oil industry are the exceptions. As often happens, the exceptions provide the greatest interest.

The record for motorcyclists is the most remarkable. Prior to 1960, the fatality rate record followed that for all road users almost precisely. This was a period when the motorcycle was the poor man's motorcar. The fatality record for all road users is dominated by that for the motorcar; so it would seem that motorcyclists were able to imitate more prosperous drivers even to the extent of maintaining a similar fatality rate.

Then, in 1960 the situation changed; motorcycling became a hazardous sport, dominated by young men for whom risks were attractive. Fatality rates have been maintained subsequently more or less at the 1960s level; there is a modest downward trend, associated no doubt with the inevitable increase in the average age of participants in the sport.

The record cannot be accounted for by the cause-and-effect theory. The transformation from cautious to reckless practice occurred in a period of less than a year, and no set of material circumstances could be so modified in such a time.

Similar arguments apply in the cases of railway passenger deaths, offshore fatal accidents and financial loss due to oil refinery accidents. The records for all these activities show an initial period of increasing fatalities or loss, culminating in a catastrophic event, following which there was a sudden drop in the fatality or loss rate. Again, this sort of record is only explicable in terms of human behaviour. It is of special interest that the same pattern of behaviour should be manifest in such different circumstances.

2.8 Scatter in fatality rate data

The wide spread of fatality rate data in aircraft and railway accidents when plotted against time was mentioned in the first part of this chapter. This wide scatter has been attributed, in part at least, to the size of the vehicle. It is certainly the case that the scatter band for road accident fatalities is much narrower. In comparative terms, the relative or proportional standard deviations are, respectively, railways: 1.0, aircraft: 0.5, and roads: 0.05.

It is concluded that the trend and direction of fatality and loss rates due to accidents; that is, whether they increase or decrease, and at what pace, are determined by the collective behaviour of the population concerned. However, in plots of fatality or loss rates as a function of time, the degree of scatter of data points is determined primarily by the material circumstances of the activity.

3 Mortality from all causes

3.1 Introduction

The justification for including a chapter on all-cause mortality in a book on fatal accidents is, in the first place, empirical. There is a most remarkable similarity between plots of male 'all-cause' mortality rates against time and those of male accident mortality for the same period and, of course, in the same country: in this case England and Wales. Bearing in mind previous findings about the relationship between accident mortality and the economic progress of nations, this relationship should not, perhaps, be too surprising. It is a matter of common knowledge that the more prosperous nations have lower mortality rates than those in an earlier stage of development. Since this rule applies likewise to fatal accidents, accidental death rates could reasonably be expected to march more or less in time with those from all causes.

Before looking at details, it is necessary to say a few words about all-cause mortality. The data to be considered here are from the English Census Office, which later became the Office for National Statistics. Records for mortality started in 1838 and, from that date, the numbers of deaths from various types of disease were recorded in an annual report on 'The Causes of Death'. In 1858 the category 'violence' was added. This category was subdivided into accident or negligence, homicide, suicide, execution and unclassified. In 1900 this system was replaced by the International Classification of Disease, which likewise contained a category for death by accident. This document has subsequently been revised at roughly 10-yearly intervals, and has become increasingly complex. The net result is that data for mortality from all causes in England and Wales are available from 1838, and for accidental death from1858.

Special interest attaches in this chapter to the relationship between mortality rates due to disease, and those resulting from accidents. For older persons, accidental death forms a very small proportion of the total, and mortality from all causes will be taken as a good approximation to mortality from disease. In the case of young people, however, such is not the case, and mortality from disease will be approximated by: (all-cause mortality minus accident mortality).

Also, a substantial proportion of accidental deaths occurred on roads, particularly in the second half of the twentieth century. As demonstrated in Chapter 1, such deaths correlate with vehicle numbers, and these vary independently of population numbers. Therefore, when looking in detail at accident mortality during the twentieth century, road deaths will be excluded from the calculation of accident mortality rates.

It is self-evident that mortality rates must vary with age, and it is customary to list mortality data according to sex and age group. For England and Wales, the early data are for 5-year groups up to age 24 and 10-year groups thereafter; more recently, 5-year groups are listed throughout.

3.2 The kinship between accident and all-cause mortalities

The similarity between plots of male accident and all-cause mortalities against time, mentioned at the beginning of this chapter, is illustrated in Figs. 3.1 and 3.2. Figure 3.1 is for the age group 20–24, and Fig. 3.2 relates to the other end of the adult age spectrum: age 65–74. The period is 1901–2000, and in both cases the upper diagram represents mortality rates from all causes, and the lower one represents accident mortality. Figure 3.1 indicates, in each case, a generally exponential fall of the rate with time, with an upward surge during each of the two war periods. In Fig. 3.2 the fall in both instances is initially somewhat irregular with much scatter but, after about 1970, settles down to a regular, non-scattered, linear drop. The detailed correspondence for these two age groups and for those below the age of 20 correspond less precisely, but all are generally similar.

It was proposed in Chapter 1 that accidents result from errors of judgement by individual human beings. As a consequence of the development of human skill, the frequency of such errors is reduced, and this is the process that regulates the observed fall of accidental deaths. Material circumstances affect the probability of an accident, but do not regulate the frequency. Their effect is a secondary one, and may influence the degree of scatter where fatal accident data are plotted against time.

A similar model may be applied to the case of death from disease. In this instance the accident is biological, not physical, but equally the frequency thereof can be reduced by the development of human skill. Thus, the risk of death from an infectious disease is reduced by improved sanitation and hygiene. Progress in surgery and medicine provides opportunities analogous to those from technology in the case of physical accidents: but again, the fall of the mortality rate is regulated by the human population.

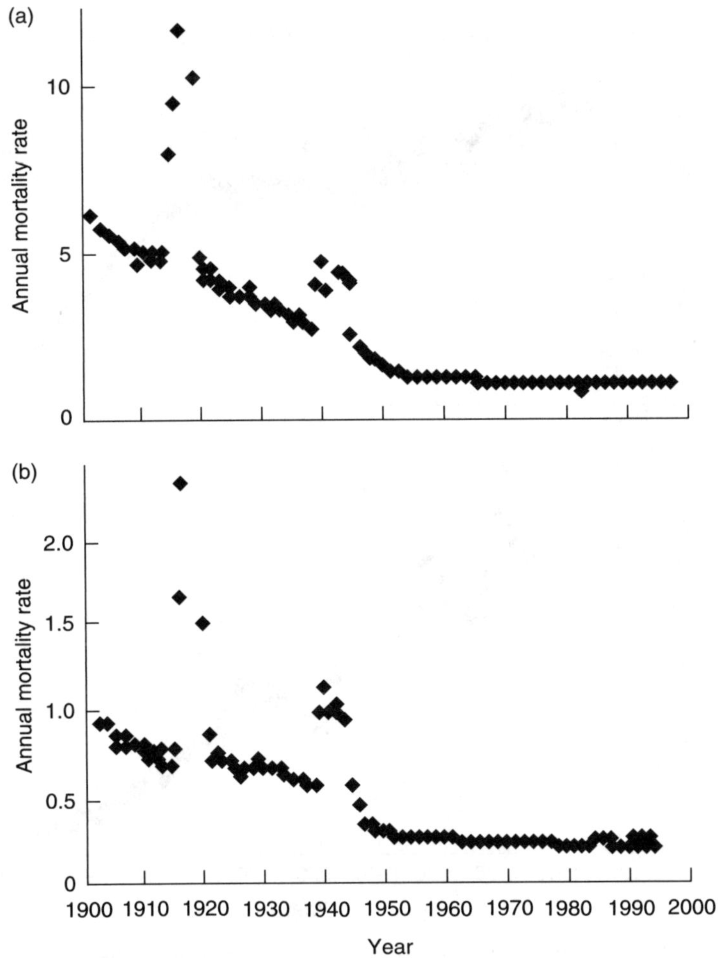

3.1 Annual mortality rates per 1000 population in England and Wales 1901–2000 (a) from all causes (b) from accidents. Male, age group 20–24. In figure (a) the high mortality rate in 1918, due to the influenza pandemic, is not shown.

Supposing the model to be correct, then the similarities of Figs. 3.1 and 3.2 would be expected. Much further evidence remains to be presented, however.

3.3 The general characteristics of all-cause mortality

The outstanding feature of the all-cause mortality record for England and Wales, and for the developed world in general, is that, during the twentieth century, death rates fell rapidly; more rapidly, it is probable, than at any

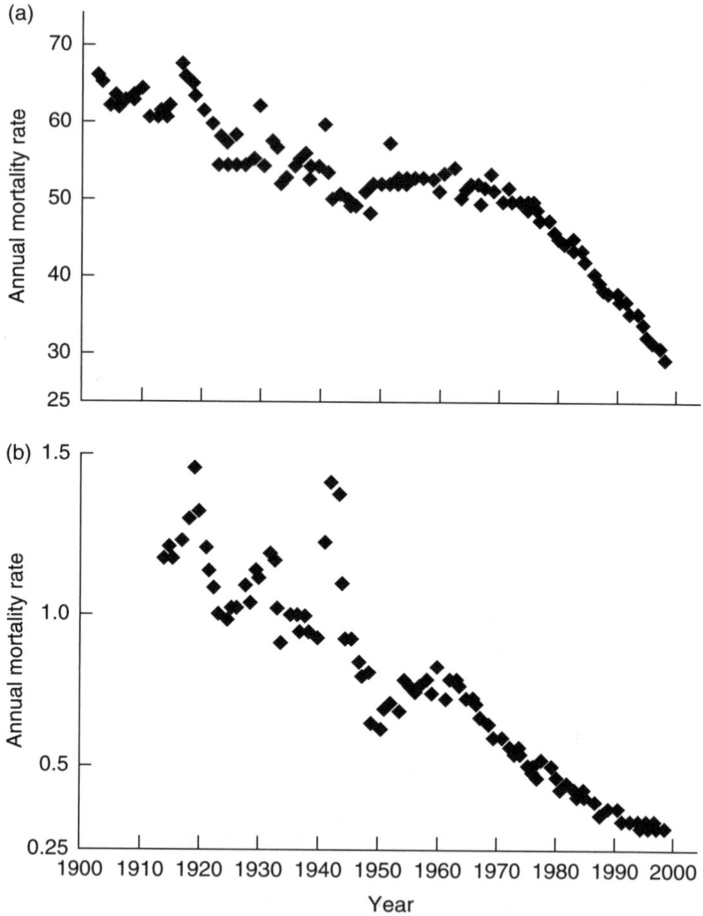

3.2 Annual mortality rate per 1000 population in England and Wales 1901–2000 (a) all causes (b) accidents. Male, age group 65–74.

time previously. This fall started during the second half of the nineteenth century. It was most rapid for infants and very young children, and least rapid for old people. The trend is generally exponential, although with many irregularities, as seen in Fig. 3.2.

The way in which all-cause mortality rates are distributed according to sex and age group is indicated in Figs. 3.3 and 3.4. Figure 3.3 shows how matters stood in 1861, while Fig. 3.4 was the position in 2000. The relative position of the sexes has not changed very much during the 140-year period. For the very young and very old, male mortality is significantly higher than female, but for intermediate age groups the difference is small. The same rule applies in the intervening years and, in plots of mortality rate against time, the data points for the two sexes follow an identical course and are close together.

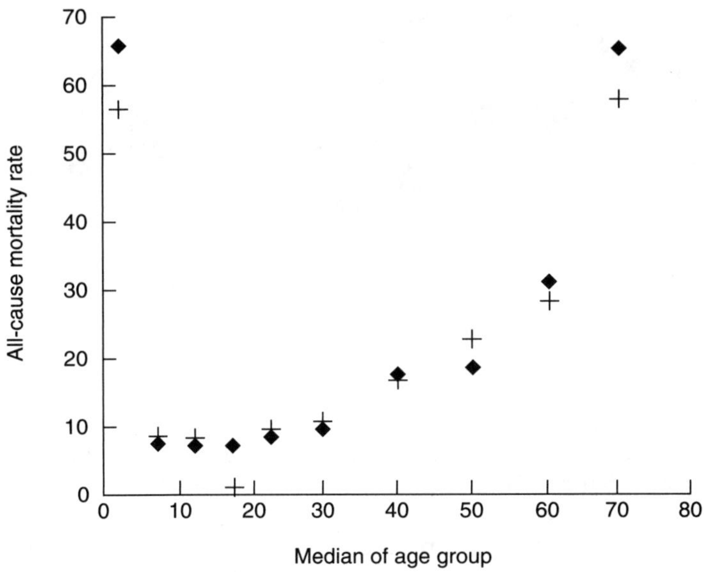

3.3 Annual mortality rate per 1000 population according to sex and age group in England and Wales in 1861. ◆ male; + female.

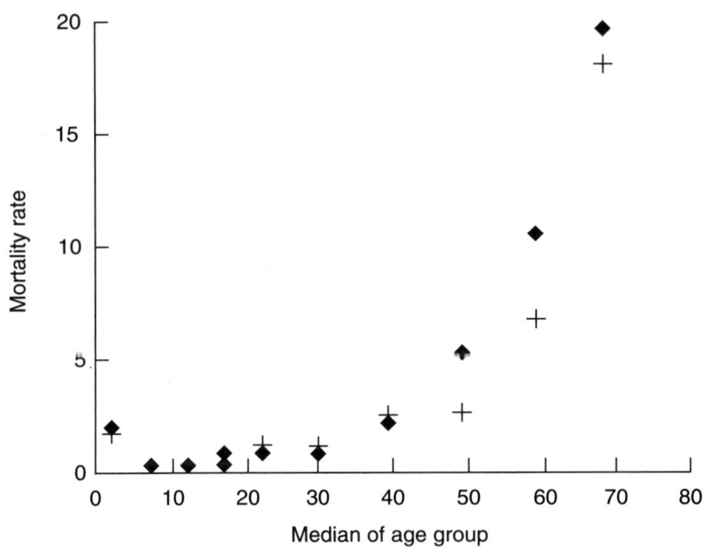

3.4 Annual mortality rate per 1000 population according to sex and age group in England and Wales in the year 2000. ◆ male; + female.

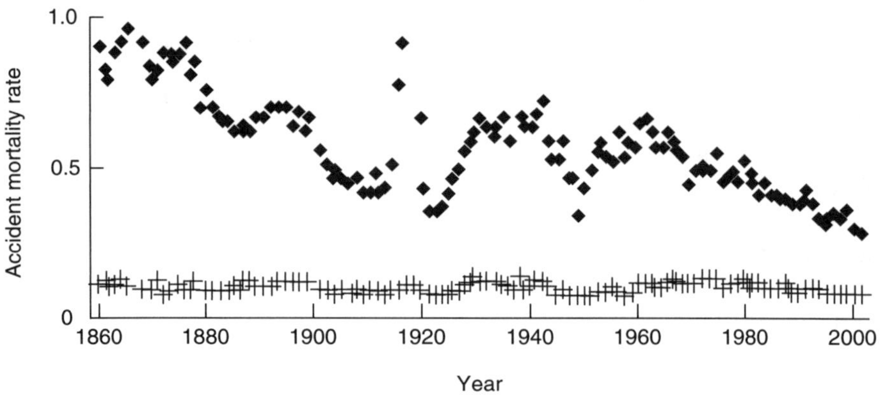

3.5 Annual death rate due to accidents per 1000 population of the 20–24 age group in England and Wales 1860–2000. Data points for 1917 (1.4) and 1918 (1.7) have been omitted. ◆ male; + female.

The other noticeable feature about Figs. 3.3 and 3.4 is the large fall in the death rates of infants and very young children from 1861 to 2000. Improvements in hygiene and obstetric care have had a dramatic effect on the probability of survival for this age group, and have greatly minimised the distress caused by deaths in childbirth and early childhood.

The equivalents to Figs. 3.3 and 3.4 for fatal accidents were shown in Figs. 1.7 and 1.8. These are similar in one respect: the reduction in accidental deaths for the very young. In the nineteenth century, numbers of babies were still-born as a result of accidental injury to the cranium or spine, and, by the year 2000, such mishaps had been largely eliminated.

In this respect the sexes were equal, but this was not the case for other age groups. Accident mortality for young men was substantially greater than that for young women; the difference has diminished with the passage of time, and it is not so great for older people.

Figure 3.5 plots male and female accident mortality rates for 20–24-year-olds in England and Wales during the period 1860–2000. The striking feature about this diagram is that the rate for females has remained virtually unchanged for 140 years. This condition is characteristic of women aged between 15 and 45; female children and older women have a higher initial fatal accident rate, which falls with time. Thus, it would seem that women of child-bearing age have a remarkable ability to avoid fatal accidents; or to put it another way, they have a consistently low level of acceptable risk. Bearing in mind the very considerable changes that have taken place in the legal, political and social status of women during the period under review, this characteristic must be genetically determined; it is an evolutionary adaptation, which must be judged as being entirely appropriate. So far as the correspondence between all-cause and accident mortalities is concerned, it would seem reasonable to regard the condition of the male as normal, and that of young women as being the exception.

A prominent feature of Fig. 3.5 is the extremely irregular character of the plot of male accident mortality rates. This was occasioned primarily by two events: war, and the appearance of the motorcar. It was recorded in Chapter 2 that the number of deaths due to road accidents started to increase in the 1930s, then fell to a low point during the war, increased afterwards to a peak in the early 1960s, and then fell again. Young men make a disproportionally high contribution to road deaths, and this is reflected in the ups and downs of the mortality rate record. These fluctuations are reproduced to a very modest degree in the female record, probably because of deaths as passengers rather than because of any attempt to emulate the male. The discrepancy between male and female accident mortality is very significant, and will be discussed in a later section.

3.4 Initiation of the fall in mortality rates

The observed fall in all-cause mortality rates during the twentieth century, which was evidently more rapid than in earlier times, naturally poses the question: how and why did it begin? The first step in attempting to answer the question is to look at the record for the nineteenth century.

The relevant data for all-cause and accident mortality are plotted in Figs. 3.6 and 3.7, for the 20 to 24 and 65 to 74 age groups. From these diagrams, and from data for other age groups, it is judged that the fall in all-cause mortality rates probably initiated in 1870, or approximately then. It is possible to establish exponential trend curves for the all-cause mortality data plots before and after 1870 and thereby obtain the annual proportional change in the rate. The results are plotted in Fig. 3.8 for age groups between ages 1 and 74. The squares are the pre-1870 data points, and crosses represent those after 1870. All the post-1870 values are negative, which means a declining rate. Pre-1870 there was a smaller declining rate for younger persons, but for older age groups the mortality rate increased with time. In later years these curves levelled and then rates began to fall as indicated in Fig. 3.2a,b. Generally, this exercise tends to confirm 1870 as a likely date for the transition to a more rapid decline in mortality from all causes.

The curves for accident mortality are more variable; they show a similar trend, but it would be difficult to assign a transition date.

3.5 The germ theory of disease

In the nineteenth and early twentieth centuries much distress was caused by the premature deaths of infants and young children, and infectious disease was, to a significant degree, responsible for this situation. Louis Pasteur, a French chemist and biologist, made a major contribution to the

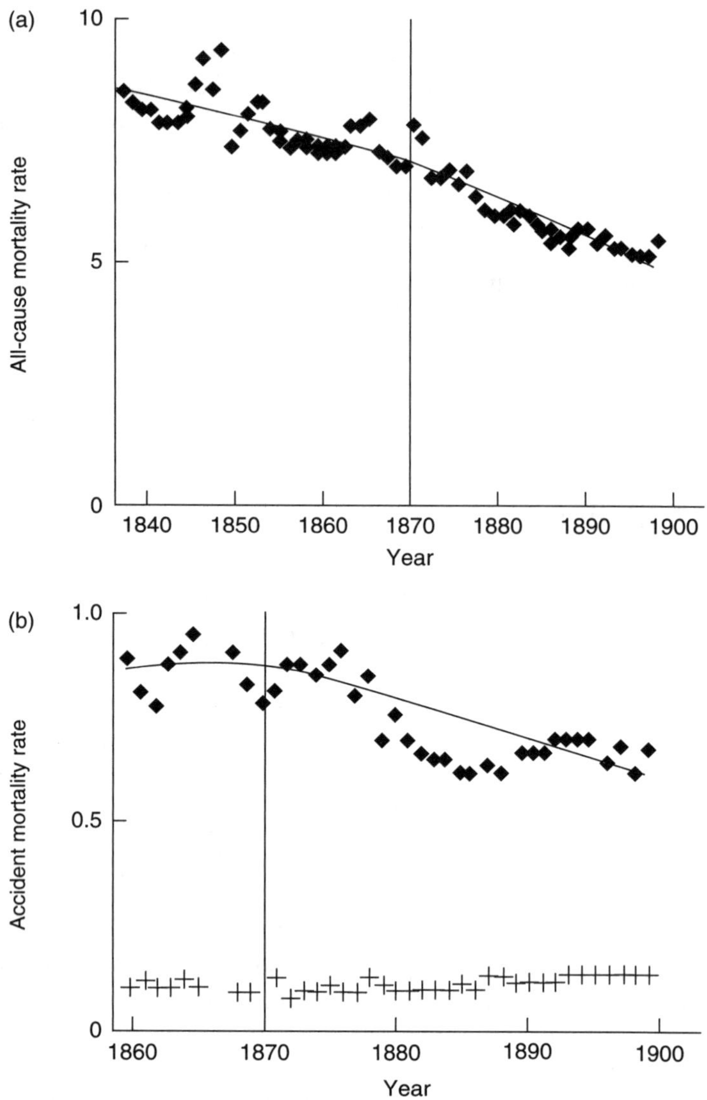

3.6 Annual mortality rate per 1000 population of the 20–24 age group in England and Wales. ◆ male; + female. (a) from all causes from 1838 to 1899 (b) due to accidents from 1860 to 1899. In Fig. 3.6 (a) ◆ represents both sexes.

understanding and, in some specific cases, to the control of the problem. Work on fermentation and on the spoilage of wine by bacterial action led to the idea that bacteria could also be responsible for some human diseases, a view that was known, at the time, as the Germ Theory of Disease. Previously, infectious disease was considered by the medical profession to be due to a miasma that rose form the surface of the Earth and in some manner

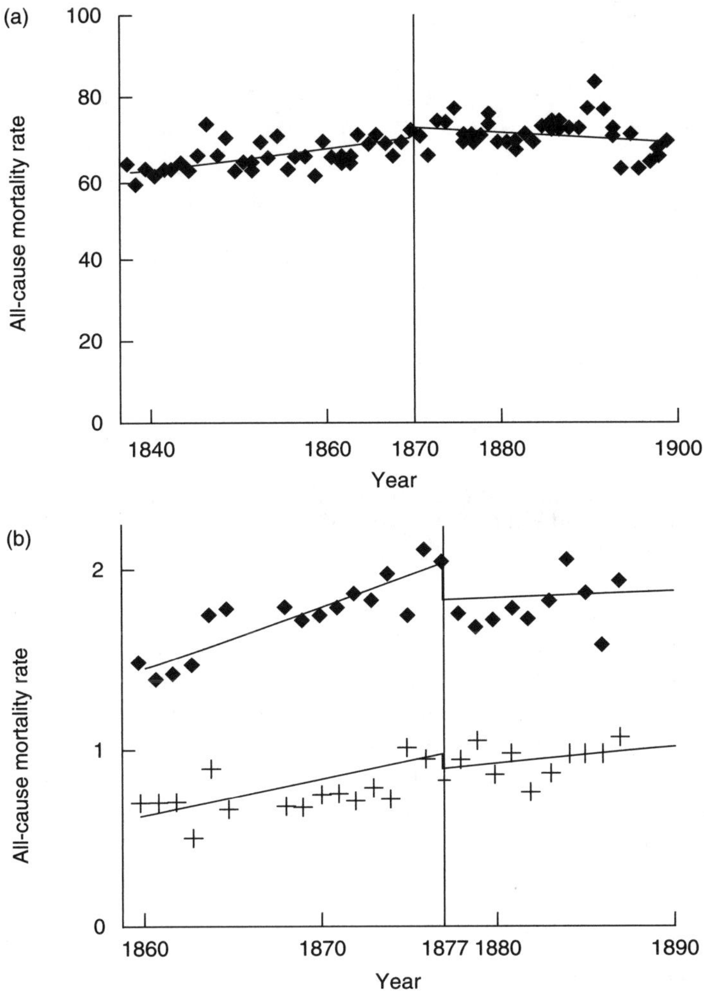

3.7 Annual mortality rate per 1000 population of the 65–74 age group in England and Wales. ◆ male; + female. (a) from all causes from 1838 to 1899 (b) due to accidents from 1860 to 1887.

invaded the body. The Miasma Theory was mystical in character, and disease so caused was not susceptible to material control. Bacteria, on the other hand, could be killed by antiseptics or evaded in one way or another, and in the 1860s Joseph Lister, a surgeon at the Glasgow Royal Infirmary, demonstrated that the sterilisation of surgical instruments using carbolic acid was effective in reducing post-operative infections.

It is highly probable that such events led to a general acceptance in Britain of the need for cleanliness and hygiene, to the widespread use of antiseptics, and to other measures that avoided the transmission of bacteria from person to person. The time scale is correct. After the initial fall in

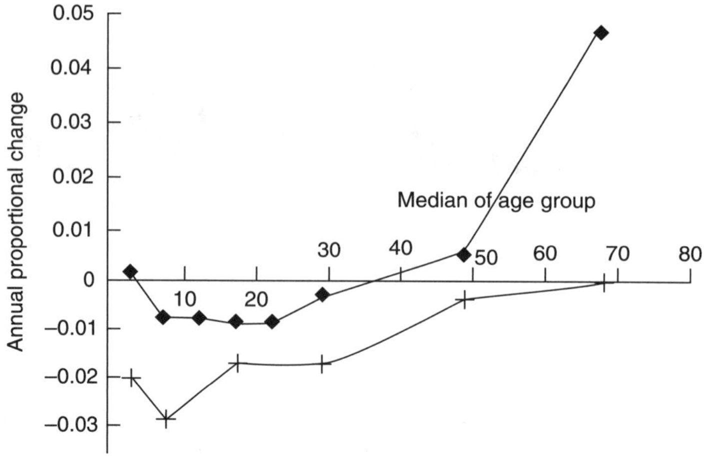

3.8 Annual proportional change of all-cause male mortality rate in England and Wales before and after 1840. ◆ from 1838 to 1869; + from 1870 to 1899.

mortality rates in 1870 (or thereabouts), there was a sharp drop in the proportion of deaths due to infectious diseases in England and Wales between 1881 and 1899. There followed a long decline such that, by 1970, death from infectious disease has become a rarity in Britain.

Thus, the general population was responsible for its own improvement in health. In the late nineteenth century the medical profession had very few effective weapons against disease, and its contribution towards this end was not significant.

It follows that the model that was developed in Chapter 1 to explain the regulated fall of accident mortality rates could also apply to mortality from disease. In this instance the essential process was the development of human skill in avoiding infection, and such was made possible by progress in science and technology. The similarity of all-cause and accident mortality records is a manifestation of their common roots.

Technology was of special importance in the defence against ineffective agents. The London sewer, which collected effluent from the whole city and discharged it at a distant point, was completed in 1860, and similar improvements were made elsewhere. Better water supplies became available, and very significant developments were made in this field during the whole of this period.

3.6 Infectious disease

Figure 3.9 is a plot of the percentage of deaths in Great Britain during the twentieth century that were due to infectious diseases, as specified in

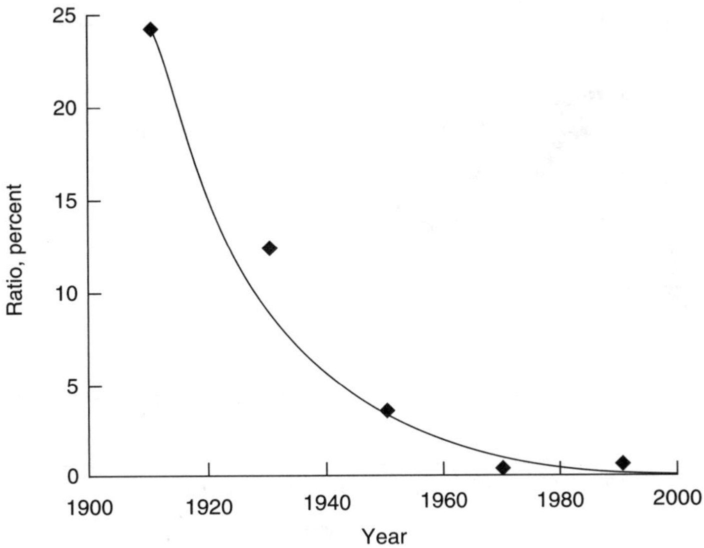

3.9 Percentage of deaths due to infectious disease in Great Britain from 1911 to 1991.

Section I of the *International Classification of Disease*. This category includes such maladies as typhus, cholera and dysentery. The fall was dramatic, and although some diseases, such as the childish infections of mumps and measles remain with us, they rarely cause death. Others have disappeared completely and their names, in the twenty-first century, are almost forgotten. Victory in this war must rank as one of the greatest human achievements of the recent past. It deserves much greater recognition, as does its guiding genius, Louis Pasteur.

3.7 Mortality rates in the twentieth century

Plots of mortality rates against time for the various age groups in England and Wales fall into two very distinct categories. The first comprises age groups 1–4 up to 35–44. Figure 3.10, for men aged 20–24, is characteristic. From 1901 to the end of the Second World War there was an exponential fall, interrupted in the case of adolescent and adult males by an upward surge during the war periods. Then, after 1946, there was a sharp drop, followed by a second exponential fall, starting at a low figure and falling at a slow pace. For the 20 to 24 age group males, this fall was at a rate of 0.34% annually, and, for children and other young adults, the pattern of events was similar. It was, of course, precisely during this period that a national health service was established in Great Britain. It would be uncharitable to suggest that increased medication caused an arrest in the

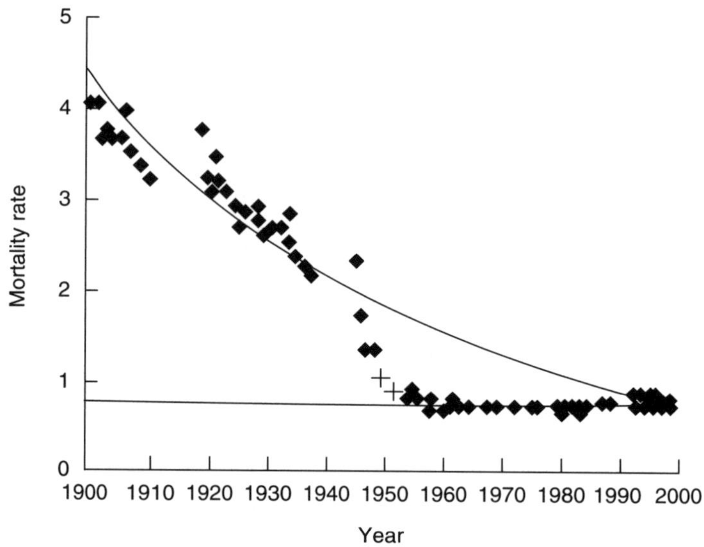

3.10 Annual mortality rate due to disease per 1000 population of the male 20–24 age group in England and Wales from 1901 to 2000. ◆ 1901 to 1949; + 1950 to 2000. Data for the two World War periods have been omitted, both in the diagram and when calculating the trend curve 1901 to 1950. The annual decline of the mortality rate is: 1901–1949, 1.5% 1950–2000, 0.34%.

improvement of the mortality rate of young people; other than resulting in a small increase of the incidence of accidental poisoning, its effect has been neutral. Medicinal treatment is, or should be, designed to improve the quality of life. The lay population had already demonstrated its ability to minimise the risk of death.

The cause of the change is, in all probability, that by 1950 the risk of death from infectious disease amongst those under the age of 45 had fallen to such a level that the room for improvement was small, and the residual disorders more intractable. A slow decrease persists, nevertheless.

Figure 3.10 was, for clarity, restricted to males. The corresponding female plot is very similar, except that in the second period, from 1954 to 2000, the mortality rate falls to an average of 0.51 per thousand population, as compared with 0.96 for males.

Figure 3.11 is the equivalent of Fig. 3.10 for the 65–74 age group, except that, in this instance, it is possible to plot data points for both sexes. This figure is characteristic of plots for all age groups between 45 and 75; it applies, in other words, to the middle-aged and the elderly.

For the period prior to 1970, there was a somewhat ragged exponential fall in mortality rate. Then, in 1970, the decline became steeper, was linear

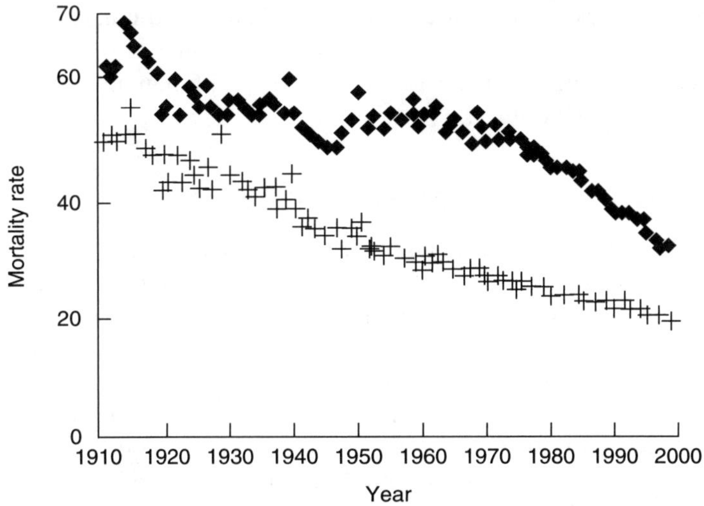

3.11 Annual mortality rate due to disease per 1000 population for the 65–74 age group in England and Wales 1911–2000. ◆ male; + female.

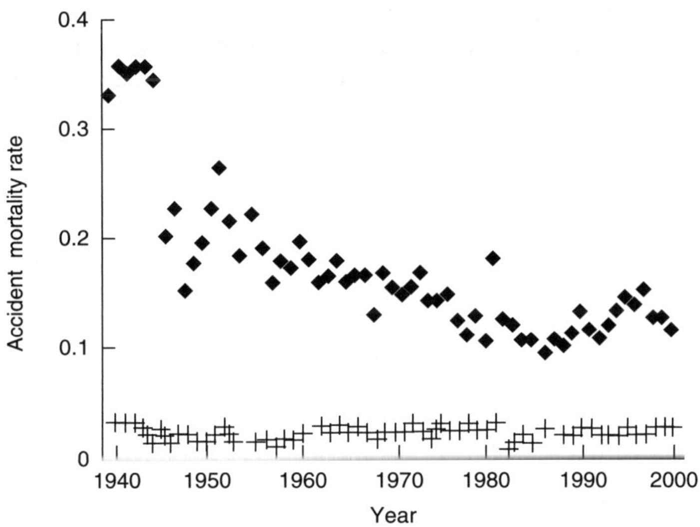

3.12 Annual mortality per 1000 population for the 20–24 age group in England and Wales due to accidents other than those on roads, 1940–2000. ◆ male; + female.

in form and showed a relatively small degree of scatter. In Fig. 3.2 it was seen that this feature also appeared in a plot of male accident mortality. Figure 3.12 shows that it is equally the case for females.

Thus, there is an indication from the mortality record of a change in behaviour of the British population in the year 1970. This change was from the relatively reckless, as evidenced by the scatter of the data points, to the relatively cautious, characterised by a steeper decline of the mortality rate and less scatter. This change is reflected in other human activities, as will be demonstrated in Chapter 4.

3.8 The influenza epidemic in 1918

The world-wide influenza pandemic, which killed more people than the 1914–1918 war, reached Britain in 1918. The worst effects were in that year but, for younger people, influenza deaths continued through 1919 and into 1920. The main interest here concerns the indications that the relevant records give about human behaviour.

1918 was, of course, a war year and the death rates both from disease and from accidents were affected; in particular, mortality rates for men were increased temporarily. To minimise the effect of this distortion, a comparison is made between the records for 1918 and those for 1917. Figure 3.13 is a plot of the ratio between all-cause mortality rates in 1918 and those in 1917 according to sex and age group. The age groups span 5 years in each plot, the oldest age group being 80–84.

The first characteristic to note about this diagram is that there is no significant difference between the sexes. In normal life the mortality rate of

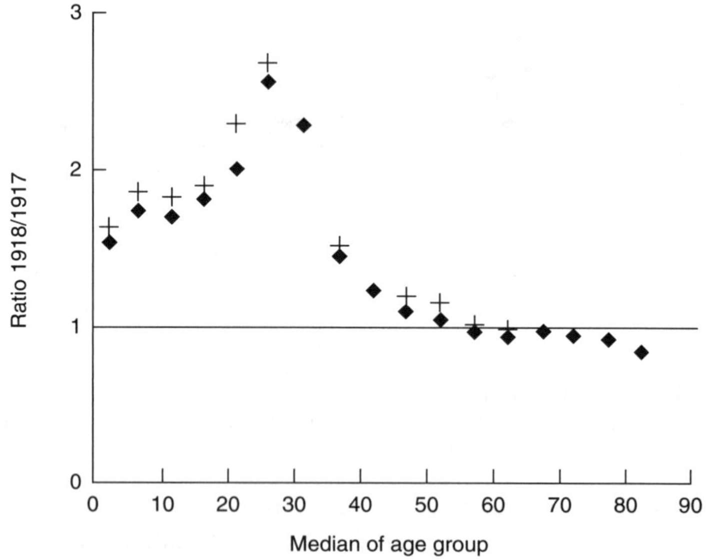

3.13 Ratio of all-cause mortality rates in 1918 and those for 1917. ◆ male; + female. Where only ◆ is shown, figures for male and female are equal.

men increases with age more rapidly than that of women, and from this (and from other indications) it could be concluded that the male is intrinsically more susceptible to disease than the female. Such, however, was not the case here, where the only significant difference between the two years was the presence in 1918 of a lethal virus. Thus, the apparent difference between the sexes in susceptibility to disease could be due to differences in behaviour. Such is indeed the case with fatal accidents, as seen in several figures, notably in Fig. 3.5.

Secondly, the age group for which the 1918/1917 ratio was highest, and which might therefore be regarded as the most susceptible to influenza, was 25–29. By the same token, the least susceptible would appear to be the very young and the very old. This is completely the opposite to conventional ideas and indeed, to common sense, and it must be concluded that Fig. 3.13 is a measure, not of susceptibility, but of the probability of infection. And this, in turn, must depend on the frequency of encounters between individuals and thus, on the activity of the age group concerned.

Finally, there is the case of those aged 55 and over. For these older people, the risk of dying in 1918 was equal to, or slightly less than, that in 1917. They would, in the normal course of events, have been less active, but it is very probable that a conscious effort was made to avoid infection; the old ones stayed indoors and remained in reasonable health.

3.9 The two World Wars

For Great Britain, the 1914–1918 and 1939–1945 wars were unique. In previous conflicts the fighting had been by a professional army but, during the two World Wars, much of the population was conscripted either for the armed services or for work directed towards their support. This total effort is reflected in the statistics for male all-cause and accidental death rates, as already observed quite frequently. It will be recalled that the increased mortality and fatality rates were amongst civilians and, although there were numbers of deaths from aerial bombardment, particularly during the Second World War, these were not sufficient to account for the upsurge.

Figures 3.14 and 3.15 plot relevant data for the 20 to 24 age group for the two war periods. The greatest increase in mortality rates was for young men between the ages of 20 and 29. The rates for women were unaffected, with the exception of the 15–19 age group, for which there was a brief and slight rise of all-cause minus accident rates during the 1914–1918 war.

In these two diagrams a comparison is made between (all-cause) mortality and accident mortality rates. The first category has been labelled 'Disease Mortality'. This is not strictly correct, because suicides and homicides have not been excluded. The consequent error is, however, very small and may reasonably be ignored. Accident mortality rates are:

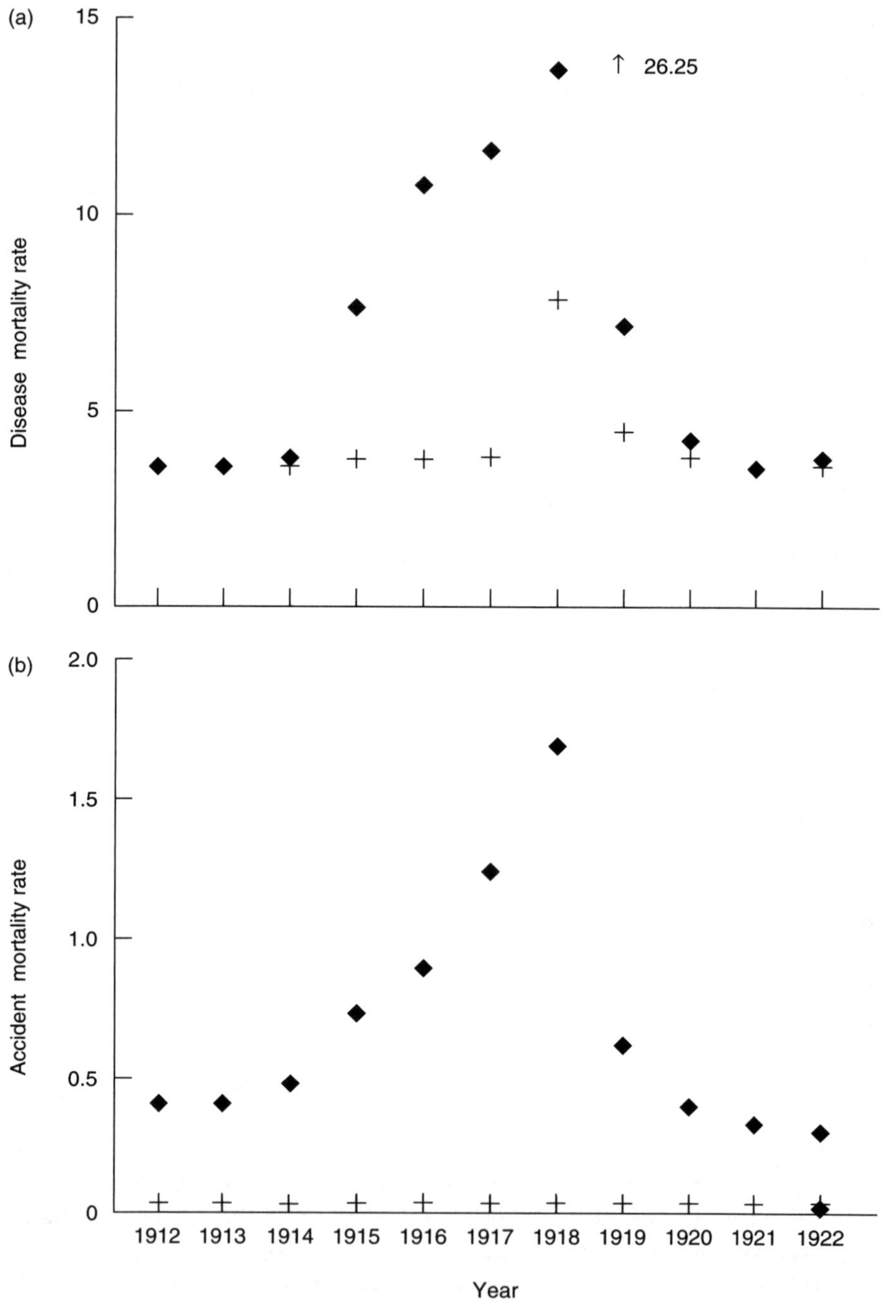

3.14 Annual mortality rate per 1000 population of the 20–24 age group in England and Wales 1912–1922 (a) due to disease (b) due to accidents, other than those on roads. ◆ male; + female.

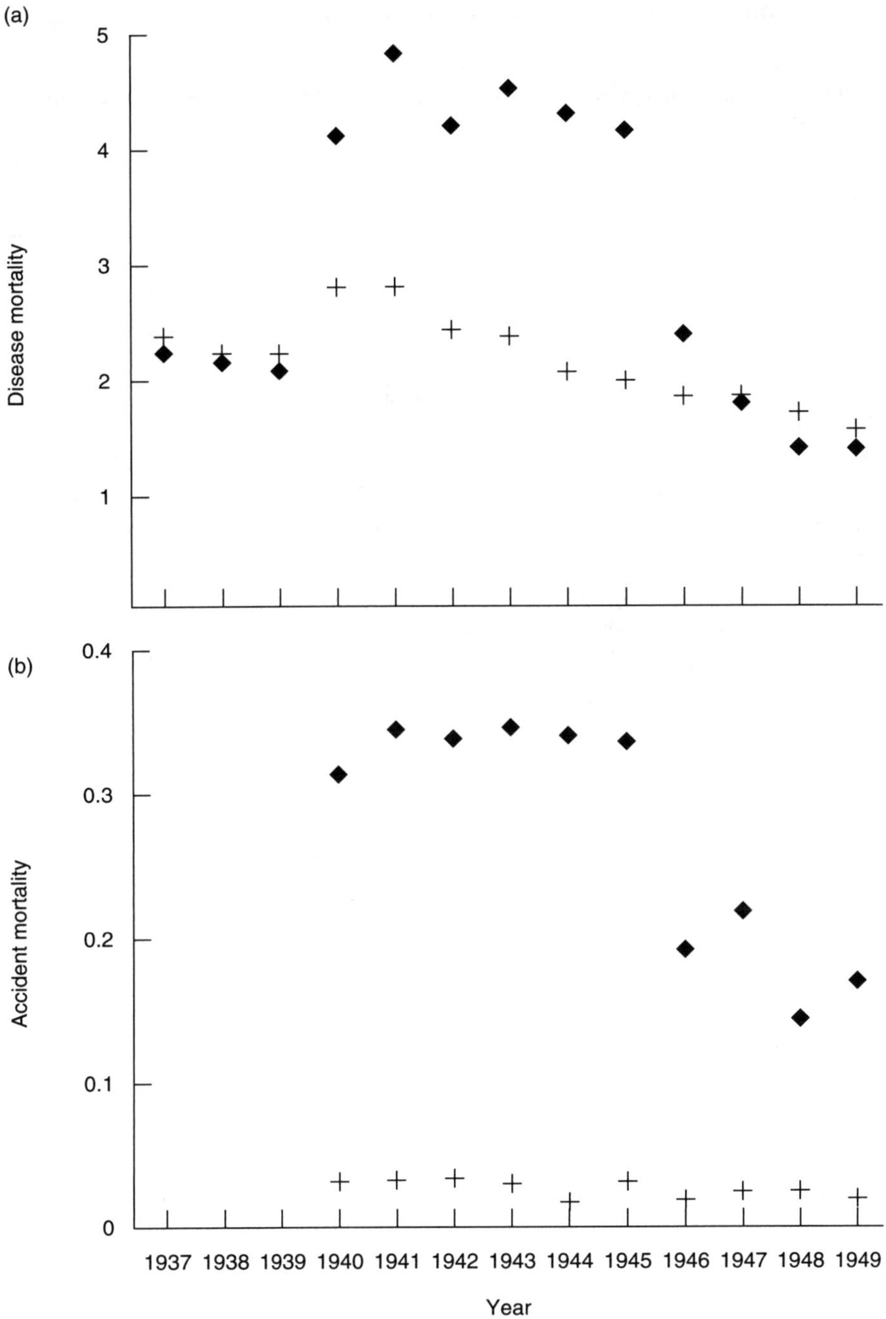

3.15 Annual mortality rate per 1000 population of the 20–24 age group in England and Wales 1937–1949 (a) due to disease (b) due to accidents, other than those on roads. ◆ male; + female.

(all accident deaths–road deaths)/population.

As already explained, this is necessary because road deaths vary with vehicle population, which in turn changes independently of the human population.

The patterns made by the data points for the two war periods are different. During the First World War the mortality rates increased steadily from 1914 to 1917, after which that due to disease rose sharply because of the influenza epidemic. During the Second World War, however, they remained almost steady from 1940 to 1945. But the patterns for disease and accidents were, in both cases, remarkably similar. Moreover, the proportional increase of male mortality rates due to disease and accidents was almost precisely the same during the First World War, and very similar during the Second. This increase has been measured as the ratio between mortality rates during the penultimate year of each war and that in 1920 and 1948, respectively. For the comparison between 1944 and 1948, road accident deaths were subtracted from the total, as before. Figures 3.16 and 3.17 display the result of these calculations.

These calculations provide evidence that the link between all-cause and accident mortalities observed in Fig. 3.1 may be quantitative in character, which adds weight to the view that these two quantities are influenced in a similar way by human behaviour.

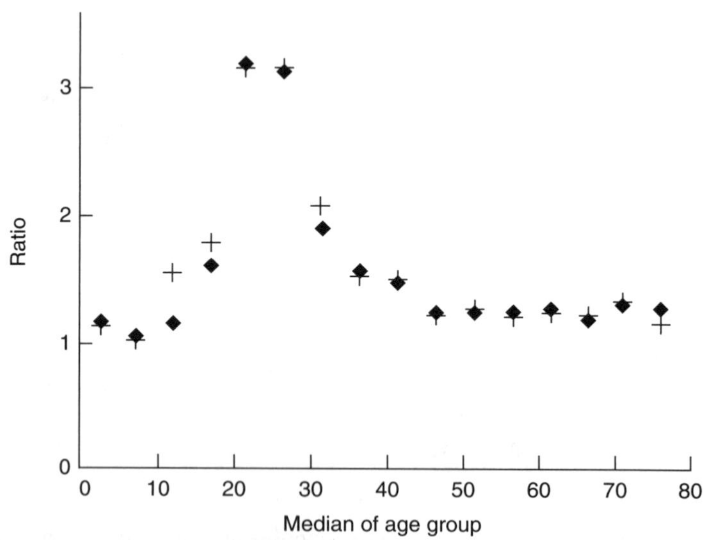

3.16 Ratio of male mortality rates for the years 1917 and 1920 for civilians in England and Wales. ◆ from disease; + due to accidents.

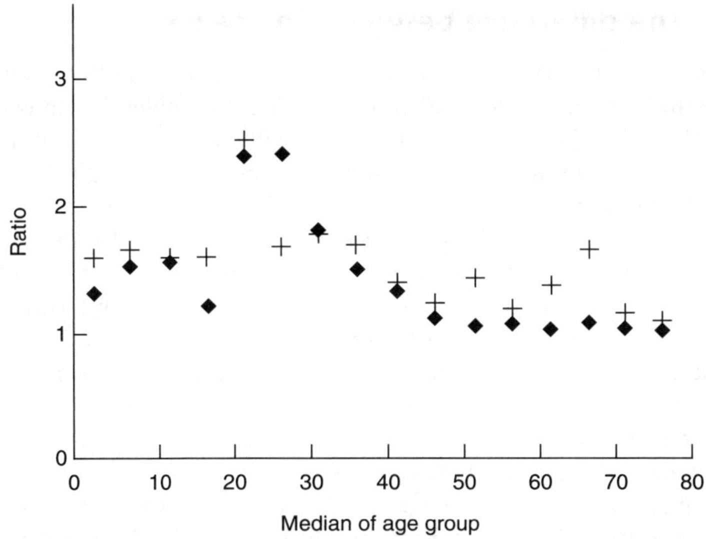

3.17 Ratio of male mortality rates for the years 1944 and 1948 for civilians in England and Wales. ◆ from disease; + due to accidents.

Regardless of theory, the rise of mortality rates of young men during the two World Wars was a very strange phenomenon. It was measured for civilians, who comprised a little less than one-third of the total population of the relevant age group. A similar acceptance of increased risk must have been the case with those engaged in the war. It was clearly of benefit to the national populations that their soldiers should, at the time of need, be prepared to accept an abnormally high level of risk. But, it is not easy to discern how this inborn characteristic should affect non-combatants. There is nothing in the factual record that would help to resolve this dilemma, and it remains a field for speculation.

One feature of the record is worth noting, however. For Great Britain, the Second World War came to life dramatically in 1940. As will be seen in Fig. 3.15, there was in that year a sharp rise in disease mortality rates. Then, in 1945, the end of the war, there was an abrupt fall both in disease and in accident mortality rates. As has been observed in other circumstances, such sudden changes cannot result from any alteration in environmental factors; they must have been caused by a change of attitude by the population of young men. It would seem that their acceptance of higher risks was switched on when the war began in earnest, and was switched off in 1945 when it ended.

3.10 The difference between the sexes

It will have been very evident from the data presented in this chapter that, other things being equal, the mortality rate for males is almost always higher than that for females. This is especially so in the case of accidents; Fig. 3.5 provides a telling example for young people of the 20–24 age group from 1860 to 2000. Accident mortality rates for women were low and almost unchanged throughout this 140-year period, whilst those for men fell exponentially from an initially high point. It has also been shown that, where such differences exist, they are highest for young adults and lowest for the very young and the very old (see, for example, Figs. 1.7 and 1.8).

A useful quantitative way to display these differences is to plot the ratio of male to female rates in accordance with the age group. This has been done for accident and all-cause mortality in Figs. 3.18 and 3.19, which are for the years 1861 and 2000, respectively.

The maximum male:female ratio for accident mortality was in 1861, when it was about 11. The corresponding figure for 2000 was 6.4; lower, but still a very substantial quantity. The ratio for all-cause mortality changed in the opposite direction. In 1861 it was close to 1 across the age spectrum: thus, in earlier times, there was little difference between the mortality rates of the two sexes.

For the year 2000, however, the plot for all causes has a similar form to that for accidents, but with a maximum of just below 3. It is possible that the virtual elimination of premature death from infectious disease has allowed an underlying tendency to appear.

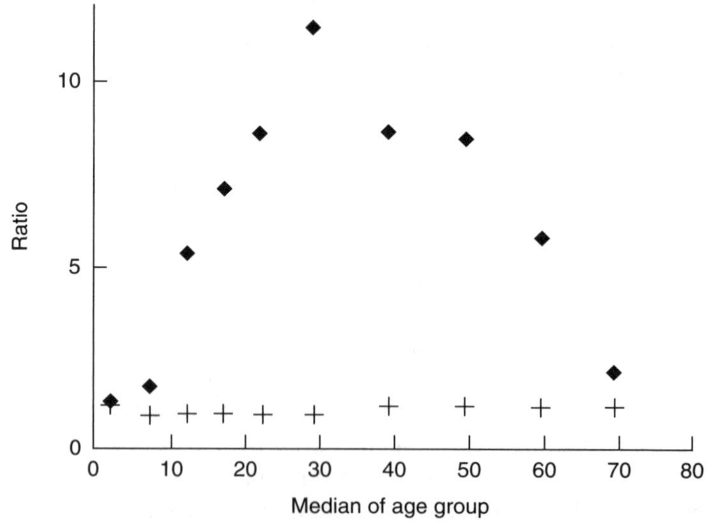

3.18 Ratio of male and female mortality rates in England and Wales in 1861. ◆ due to accidents; + from all causes.

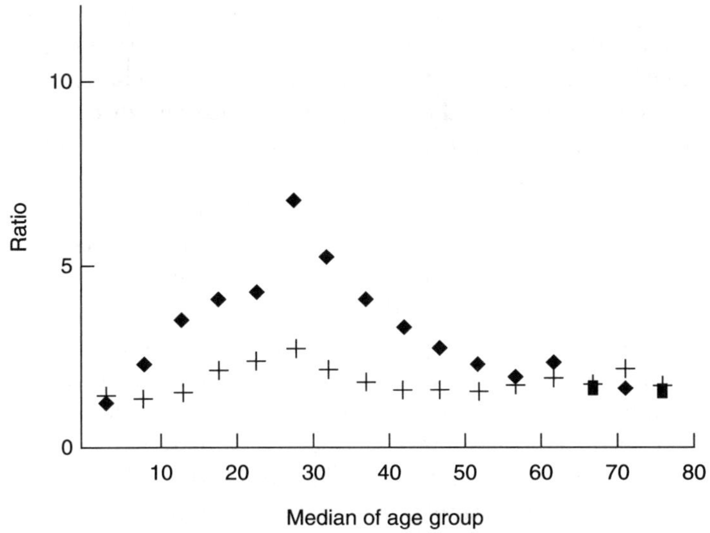

3.19 Ratio of male and female mortality rates in England and Wales in the year 2000. ◆ due to accidents; + from all causes.

3.11 Comment

The justification for including a chapter on mortality from all causes in a book concerned with fatal accidents is primarily empirical; based in the first place on the similarity between plots of accident and all-cause mortality versus time, as exemplified in Figs. 3.1 and 3.2. However, it is also in accordance with a general view of the fall of accident mortality rates that has occurred during the twentieth century, namely that it has been regulated by the human population. If such is the case for accidents, then it should be equally applicable to death from other causes. There is, of course, a common incentive for the reduction of mortality rates: that is, for the preservation of life.

It is natural for humans to believe that their affairs are directed by a superior authority of some sort. However, when mortality rates in Britain started to fall in the latter part of the nineteenth century, no such authority existed. Medical doctors had only a small number of effective drugs, and treatments were, for the most part, ineffectual. Mortality rates for children and young people fell rapidly during the first half of the twentieth century, when effective medical treatment was lacking, and then fell relatively slowly during the second half after 1950, when effective drugs became available. In the case of older persons, mortality rates started to fall sharply in 1970. In neither instance was there any correlation between the decline of morality rates and the effectiveness of medical practice.

Thus, the British population continues to regulate its mortality risk. On the other hand, the application of scientific method in medicine has cured many complaints and alleviated suffering. There is a dilemma here, which it is possible to resolve by a principle already established, namely that technological developments make human progress possible, but that the human population concerned determines the pace and discretion thereof.

Regardless of such theoretical notions, there is one feature of the record that deserves comment: the increase of both accident and all-cause mortality rates amongst young men during the two major wars of the twentieth century. It was found that the proportional increase in the rate was the same for accident as for all-cause mortality in both wars, and this provides strong support for the linkage between these two quantities.

It seems probable that this phenomenon reflects a reaction on the part of young men to a threat to national sovereignty. It must be an inherent characteristic; one which has evolved in response to similar threats stretching far back in time. Women have not been so affected.

There is one detail that may be significant. During the First World War, accident and all-cause mortality rates both increased progressively. In the second conflict, however, they rose sharply in 1940 and then stayed more or less at the same level until after 1945. At the beginning of the 1914–1918 war, Great Britain was the most powerful country in the world; at least, such was the opinion of most citizens. As the war progressed, it must have become apparent that this was an illusion, and the perceived threat must have correspondingly increased. In the Second World War, however, the threat of invasion suddenly became a reality in 1940, and there were no illusions to be eroded.

Finally, the difference between the sexes must be considered. Figure 3.5 shows how accident mortality rates changed for those aged from 20 to 24 between 1860 and the end of the twentieth century. The large initial gap between male and female plots has diminished with time, such that the ratio between male and female rates, which was 11 in 1861, had fallen to 7 in the year 2000. For younger and older persons the discrepancy is less, but is still there.

Now the accident mortality rate may reasonably be regarded as a measure of the degree of risk that is acceptable to the people in question. Also, a higher mortality rate is indicative of more reckless behaviour, and vice versa. Thus, in England and Wales, male and female differ very substantially in their attitude to risk, and there is no reason to suppose that Britain is unique in that respect. Acceptance of risk results in higher accident mortality, but it also has benefits. Taking decisions can be risky. Pioneering, whether of the physical or the intellectual kind, is always risky. So, of course, is the life of a soldier. The sexes are demonstrably unequal, and it is most beneficial that this should be the case.

4
Economic growth

4.1 Introduction

At the beginning of this book it was demonstrated that there exists an inverse relationship between economic growth and fatal accident rates, such that the more prosperous countries have lower accident mortality rates and that, for a particular nation (Great Britain), accident mortality rates fell as national productivity increased. It is considered that such relationships exist because both quantities reflect human development as a whole, and that the connection is innate, not fortuitous.

It is relevant, therefore, to consider the records relating to economic growth, since they may throw some light on how human behaviour affects safety and how, in specific cases, the inverse relationship applies.

The most useful measure of economic growth is the quantity that is known in Britain as the 'per capita gross domestic product', and which may be specified in this book as 'national output per head' or 'national productivity'. This quantity may be calculated in three ways:

- as the sum of all wages and salaries of those engaged in productive work
- as the total expenditure
- or as the total value of all goods produced

in each case divided by the number of resident citizens. Precise agreement between these measurements is not to be expected, and a compromise figure may be adopted.

The per capita gross domestic product may be expressed in terms of current price, or at constant prices. The first figure results from, for example, summing wages and salaries at their contemporary value. Constant price figures are obtained by dividing those for currencies by a price index, which is a measure of the price of a standard range of goods at any particular time. The constant price figure provides a true measure of the economic growth or decline and will invariably be used here. In most instances the per capita gross domestic product will be expressed in terms of the value of the pound sterling in the year 2000, shown as '£2000'.

Figures are taken from the *Cambridge Economic Survey*, which, for Great Britain, covers the period 1855–1983. These have been updated by data supplied by the Office for National Statistics in London.

Figure 4.1 shows how the national output per head has increased in Great Britain from 1858 to 2000. In this diagram the data points are plotted at 5-year intervals so as to eliminate unnecessary detail and to clarify general trends. The increase in prosperity has been exponential in character. It took place in two phases. During the first period, from 1858 to 1950, there was an average annual increase very close to 1%. After 1950, there was an abrupt change; the annual increase doubled to 2%. During both periods, data points conformed very closely to the trend curve. As will be seen later, an annual plot presents a less well-ordered picture.

Figure 4.2 is the corresponding plot for accident mortality in England and Wales. It has been noted that the figures for England and Wales provide a good approximation to those for the country as a whole, so these two diagrams may reasonably be compared on equal terms.

Indeed, Fig. 4.2 provides a mirror image of Fig. 4.1. The plot is once again exponential, but the mortality rate decreases with time, in conformity with the inverse relationship established earlier. Moreover, the exponential fall occurs in two phases. During the first phase the annual decrease was 0.55%, whilst during the second phase it was 1.5%. The correspondence was almost precisely quantitative in character.

It is evident that, in 1950, there was a very significant change in human behaviour. Previously, in Chapter 2 particularly, where casualty or loss rates have reached a peak, and have then fallen precipitously, such phe-

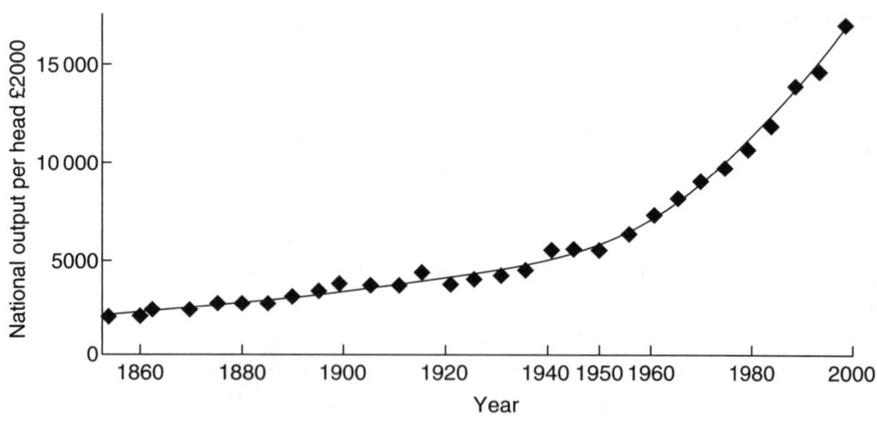

4.1 Annual national output per head of Great Britain in terms of the pound sterling at its value in the year 2000, 1855–2000. Annual growth rate: 1855–1949: 1%, 1950–2000: 2%.

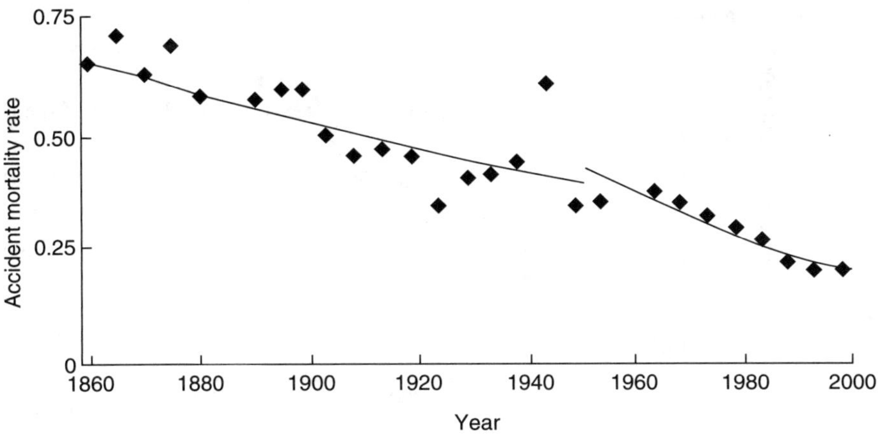

4.2 Accident mortality rate per 1000 population in England and Wales 1860–2000. Annual fall of mortality rate: 1860–1949, 0.55%; 1950–2000, 1.5%.

nomena were attributed to a change of attitude by the population concerned. In response to the threat of an increasing hazard, behaviour changes from relatively reckless to relatively cautious. In the present instance no such ready explanation is available. The war was at an end, but the danger of nuclear war with Russia remained, and the peace was not a tranquil one. It must be recognised, therefore, that a spontaneous, self-generated change of human behaviour is possible. The change from a rising to a falling trend for road casualties in Great Britain recorded in Chapter 1, and attributed there to concern about increased road deaths, may likewise have been spontaneous.

4.2 Economic growth in Britain: details

The annual plot of national output per head for Great Britain is very much less smooth than the 5-year plot of Fig. 4.1. It is best divided into three phases: 1855–1899; 1900–1949; and 1950–2000. As indicated in Fig. 4.1, the growth rate for the first two periods was almost the same: 1.06% and 0.92% annually, respectively, whilst in the third period it was 2.1%. The scatter of data was very much greater in the second period than in the other two, the relative standard deviations being 0.026, 0.082 and 0.027.

Data for these three periods are plotted annually in Figs. 4.3, 4.4 and 4.5, respectively. The span of the vertical scale in these three diagrams is necessarily different, and this may give a false visual impression. Thus, Fig. 4.5 appears to be a much smoother plot than Fig. 4.3, but the proportional scatter is very similar for both.

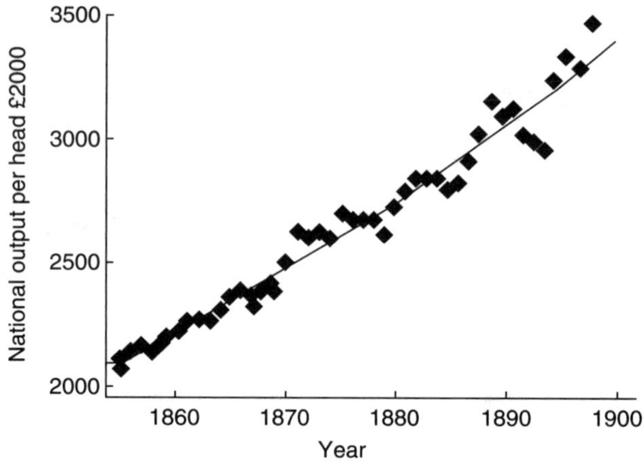

4.3 Annual national output per head in Great Britain in terms of the pound sterling at its value in the year 2000, 1855–1899.

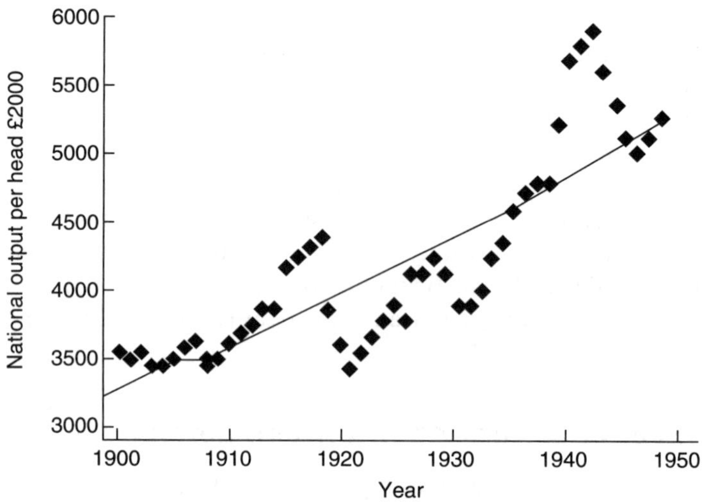

4.4 Annual national output per head in Great Britain in terms of the pound sterling at its value in the year 2000, 1900–1949.

There is a truly remarkable symmetry shown by these plots. For the first half of the twentieth century, there was a serious distortion resulting from the two wars which in turn resulted from political instability in Europe. Records for the first half of the nineteenth century are lacking: were they available, there would almost certainly have been a similar disturbance due to the Napoleonic wars, which likewise were caused by political instability in Europe. The second half of both centuries saw periods of relative peace,

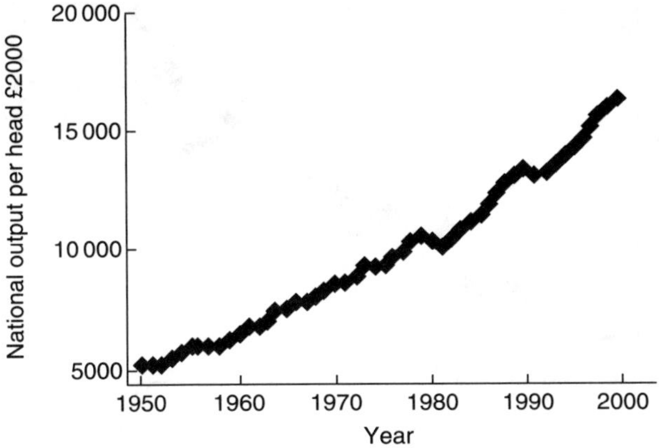

4.5 Annual national output per head in Great Britain in terms of the pound sterling at its value in the year 2000, 1950–2000.

with a corresponding low degree of scatter in the economic record. Then, towards the end of both centuries, there was a serious recession. In the first, in 1891, there was a loss of output of 5.2%; in the second, in 1989, the fall was 1.7%.

4.3 Boom and slump

A notorious feature of productive activity in the nineteenth and twentieth centuries was the tendency for a period of increasing prosperity to end in a sudden collapse, causing bankruptcies, unemployment, financial loss and general distress. These periodic slumps were superimposed on a generally rising trend and did not affect the pace of increase to any significant extent.

A similar condition was encountered in Chapter 2, with records for fatal accidents in operating mobile craft used in oil and gas exploration, and in the case of financial loss due to accidents in oil refineries. In both cases fatality and loss rates rose to a peak, followed by a precipitous fall. Moreover, these falls occurred at about the same time as there were economic recessions in Western European countries. The implied connection is not so far-fetched as it might appear at first sight. In both instances there is a change in human behaviour from relatively reckless to relatively cautious. With economic growth, however, this alternation continues. Moreover, the change in behaviour is progressive, not sudden, and when the relevant data are plotted against time, they form a roughly sinusoidal form. Figure 4.6 shows the plot of national output per head in Britain for the second half of the nineteenth century, where a perturbation of sinusoidal form and increasing amplitude has been added to the trend curve. This

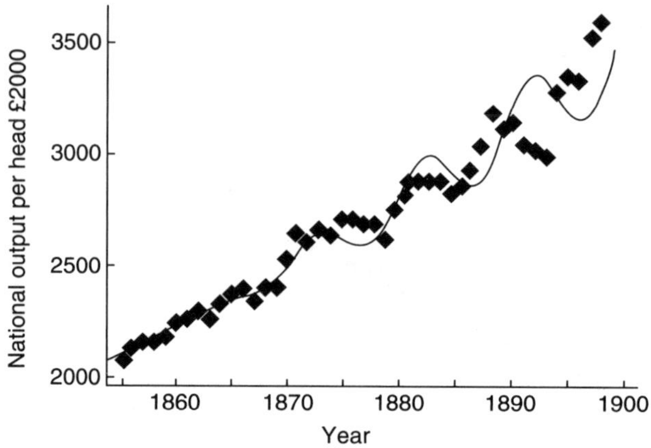

4.6 Annual national output per head in Great Britain in terms of the pound sterling at its value in the year 2000, showing a trend curve with sinusoidal perturbations of increasing amplitude.

represents the data reasonably well except for the final boom and slump, where the fluctuations took place in a shorter time. The final slump was severe, resulting in a 5% fall in output, and there was much distress amongst those people who were put out of work.

Subsequently, economic growth resumed, and merged into the boom that preceded the First World War.

Very sharp reductions of fatal accident rates were recorded for some of the activities surveyed in Chapter 2. The tendency for more gradual change in the case of economic growth rates indicates that there is an element of inertia in this process. The national output per head, which is the measure of economic growth, is the final outcome of a great multitude of transactions between individuals and of contributions to the production of food and goods, and this leviathan is unlikely to change speed quickly.

The record of economic growth in the second half of the twentieth century gives a plot similar to that for the second half of the nineteenth century; its deviations from the trend curve are sinusoidal in form with an amplitude increasing with time and culminating in a severe slump. However, as noted earlier, the proportional fall in 1989 was much smaller than in 1891, and the amplitude of the preceding undulations was corresponding less. This diminution in the swing from boom to slump is in line with the general diminution of the acceptability of risks.

4.4 The War period: 1900–1950

It may be recalled from Chapter 2 that there was an uncharacteristic rise in the fatal accident rate of British manufacturing industry during the years before the outbreak of war in 1914. This rise may, in fact, have been one of the precursors of the First World War.

In the early years of the twentieth century there was much concern in Great Britain about the increase in size of the German navy. Ever since the Battle of Trafalgar in 1805, the British navy had enjoyed an undisputed superiority over all others, and this position had been underpinned by technological developments such as bulk steel and the steam turbine. There was a determination to maintain this state of affairs, and the country therefore embarked on a large programme of naval re-armament. This activity affected the whole of manufacturing, where the numbers employed rose steadily. It is very possible that the combination of boom conditions and self-evident preparations for war was a stimulus for the change in attitude, which led to a higher rate of fatal accidents.

It has been proposed by those who consider such matters, that the two World Wars of the twentieth century really represented two phases of a single conflict. In the 1914–1918 war the machine gun gave the defence such an over-riding advantage that a decisive conclusion was impossible. Thus, there was an armistice, after which, following a long period of recovery, the combatants regrouped, re-armed and continued the struggle. The intervening period was one of considerable scientific and technological advance, but, possibly because of the political uncertainty and instability in Europe, this was not matched by corresponding economic change.

The record for economic productivity in Britain would appear to support this view. During the intervening war period, the rate of improvement was no greater than during the nineteenth century, and it was interrupted by a recession in the 1930s. Then, after 1945, when there was a decisive end to the conflict, the annual rate of increase of the per capita gross domestic product doubled to 2%, and a period of confident economic progress ensued.

Indeed, the economic records for the two World Wars, as far as Great Britain is concerned, are remarkably similar. The wartime economies provided a regulated succession of boom and slump. There is a steady rise in output during an initial period when factories are adapted to the production of war material; this rises to a peak, then falls at the end of the War to a low point as factories re-adjust to peacetime activities. This general pattern obtained for both World Wars, but there are interesting differences, as shown in Fig. 4.7. Firstly, the peak in production for the First World War was in 1918, the year of the final German offensive and then the armistice. In the Second World War this peak occurred in 1943, two years before the end. In fact, 1943 was a turning point in the Second World War; and in that year it became apparent that a German defeat was inevitable. In Britain, the motorcar population started to rise: a sure sign of confidence.

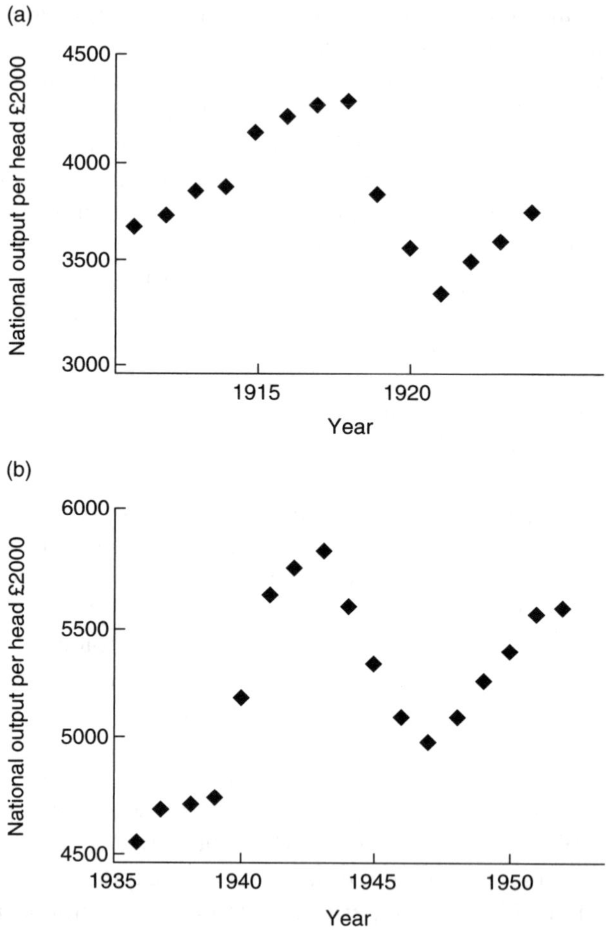

4.7 Wartime boom and slump: national output per head in terms of the pound sterling at its value in the year 2000 in Great Britain shortly before, during, and shortly after the two World Wars (a) 1911–1924 (b) 1936–1952.

Secondly, at the bottom of the depression that followed the First World War, the per capita gross domestic product was 16% below the 1913 figure. A similar comparison for the Second World War shows an *increase* of 5%. It is very likely that the post-1918 depression, which initiated a period of mass unemployment, particularly amongst industrial workers in the north of England, was a direct consequence of the pre-War rearmament boom. No such boom occurred before 1939: Britain was dragged reluctantly, and none too well prepared, into the Second World War.

It will be apparent that the plots of national output per head for the two World Wars bear a fair degree of similarity with those for the mortality rates of young civilian men during the same period.

Accordingly, Figs. 4.8 and 4.9 compare national productivity with accident mortality rates for civilian men 20 to 24 years old during both war periods.

The correspondence proves to be very close. The paired plots show not only a similar trend, but peak in the same year and, after 1943, show a similar post-war depression followed by recovery.

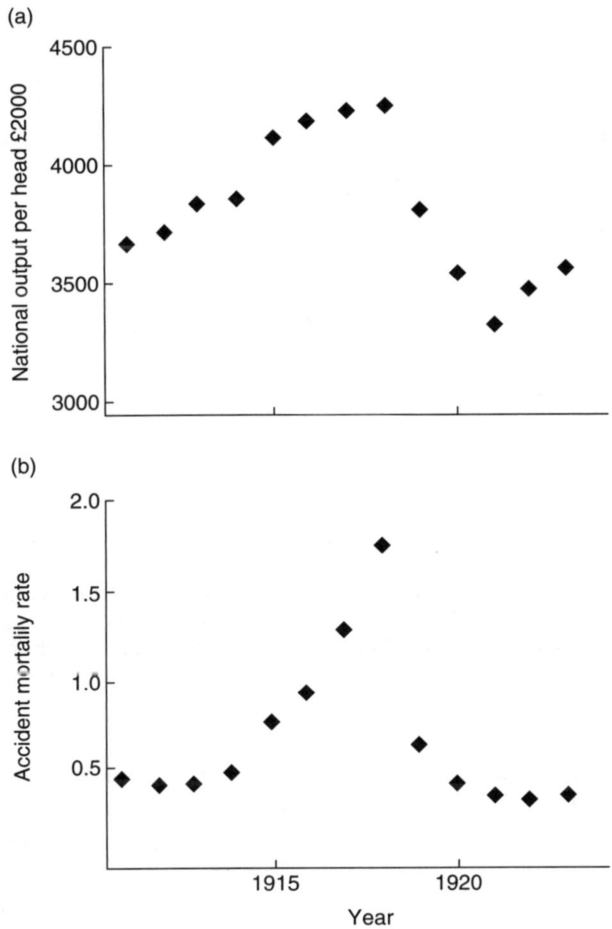

4.8 Comparison between (a) the national output per head for Great Britain and (b) the accident mortality rate per 1000 population of the civilian male 20–24 age group in England and Wales for the period 1911–1923.

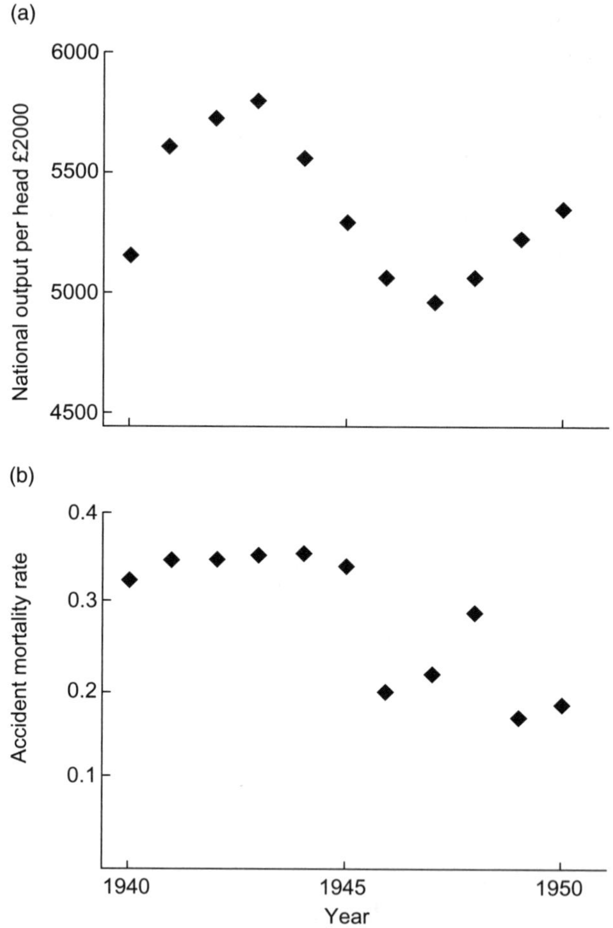

4.9 Comparison between the national output per head for Great Britain and the mortality rate per 1000 population of the civilian male 20–24 age group in England and Wales due to accidents other than those on roads, 1940–1950 (a) national output per head (b) accident mortality rate.

It may be recalled that, for young men, all-cause mortality rates also increased during the war periods, and that this increase was proportionally similar to that for accident mortality rates in general (for young men only, of course).

One of the features of fatality rates due to road accidents in Great Britain, as recorded in Chapters 1 and 2, is that, when plotted against time, data points for the period after the Second World War fall precisely on the same trend curve as that for the pre-war period, in spite of an upsurge in road death rates during the war. This continuity, it has been suggested, occurred because the wartime upsurge was due to a minority of drivers

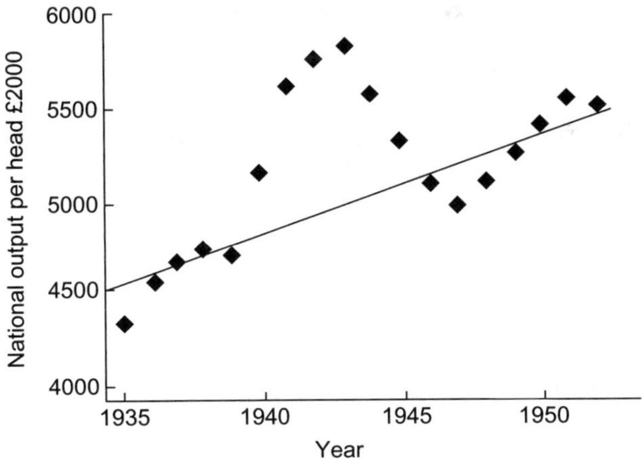

4.10 National output per head for Great Britain 1934–1952, showing continuity of trend in annual output before and after the Second World War.

(young men, of course) and that the majority continued along the normal trend of falling rates. At the end of the war, the reckless ones conformed with the majority, and the trend of fatality rate reduction continued as before.

Data for economic growth before and after the Second World War show similar characteristics, although, in this case, the trend is upwards. Figure 4.10 shows the relevant data points and trend curve. During the war only a proportion of the population was engaged directly on the production of weapons and munitions; most people continued in their peacetime activities, even if the circumstances were not very comfortable. Thus, the normal rate of growth prevailed.

These circumstances did not obtain before and after the First World War, because of the height of the pre-war boom and the depth of the post-war depression.

4.5 The 1930s Depression

The slump that occurred in the United States and in the countries of Western Europe in the 1930s was quite different in character from those of 1891 and 1989. It was initiated by a much-publicised collapse of prices on the stock exchange in New York. The shock of this event caused a widespread loss of confidence in America and in Europe, leading in turn to a slow-down of productive activity.

Figure 4.11 is a plot of the gross national output of the USA and of Great Britain from 1925 to 1938. The figures are at constant prices and are shown

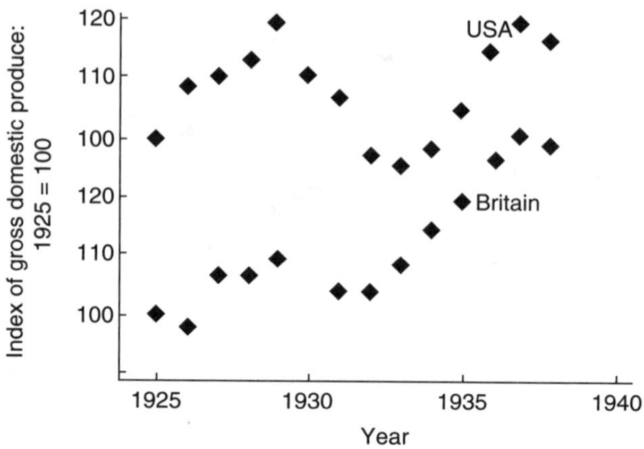

4.11 The effect of the 1929 Wall Street stock market collapse on the index of gross national domestic product of the USA and on that of Great Britain, 1925–1938. In both cases the index for the year 1925 was set at 100. The upper set of data are for the USA.

as an index, with that for 1925 being set at 100. In this diagram the upper set of data is for America and the lower one is for Great Britain.

There are two features to note. Firstly, as with other economic recessions, the pattern of data points indicates a gradual, rather than a precipitate change. Secondly, the proportional loss of output and the duration of the slump were much less severe in Britain than in the USA. The percentage loss in output from 1928 to the lowest point was just below 7% for Britain and about 20% in the USA. And the durations (that is to say, the times taken to return to the pre-slump level of productivity) were 5 years in Britain and 8 years in the USA.

Evidently, the shock effect of the 1929 Wall Street calamity was somewhat attenuated in crossing the Atlantic. Of the European nations, Germany, which suffered a loss of 9% in output in 1929, probably fared worst.

The international character of the economic downturn should not be surprising. In Chapter 2 much of the fatality and loss data are for international operations, and most of these activities, exploration for oil and gas, for example, share a common technology. Traditionally, national economies have been very different, but in the twentieth century they became increasingly interdependent.

4.6 Price inflation in Britain 1900–2000

In Great Britain, as in other developed countries, prices rose during the twentieth century; somewhat raggedly at first, but, in the last 30 years, in a more dramatic fashion. Figure 4.12 is a plot of the price index for Great Britain from 1900 to the year 2000, the figure for the final year being set at 100.

The price rise is in two phases. In the first, from 1900 to 1970, the increase was generally exponential. Then, from 1970 to 2000, it became linear, with a steeper gradient. There is a short transition period between these two phases.

Figure 4.13 shows the initial period in more detail. From 1900 to 1907 prices were unchanged. Then, in the years prior to the First World War, they started to rise to a peak in 1918, after which they fell sharply. The inter-war years were deflationary, with a slow fall. Then, during the Second World War and until 1970, prices resumed their exponential rise. The solid line in Fig. 4.13 is the exponential trend curve.

Inflation is commonly measured as the annual percentage change in the price index. This quantity has been calculated for the data plotted in Fig. 4.13, and the results are shown in Fig. 4.14. Other data have indicated that Britain suffered a severe economic shock following the First World War; these figures, which indicate a maximum inflation rate of nearly 30% during the war, followed by negative inflation (deflation) at –18.5% in 1921, confirm that there was indeed a catastrophic decline.

Subsequently, up to the 1960s, the inflation rate was more or less constant, which is consistent with the generally exponential trend of price increases.

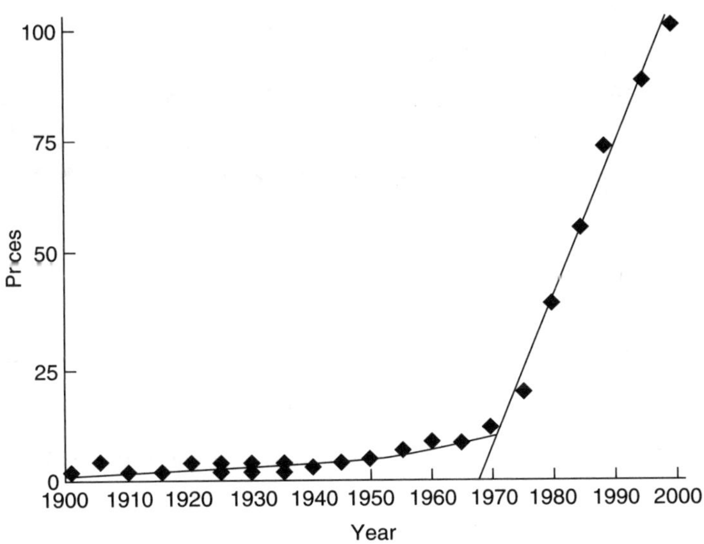

4.12 Index of prices in Great Britain 1900–2000. The index figure for 2000 = 100. The change from exponential to linear inflation occurred in 1970.

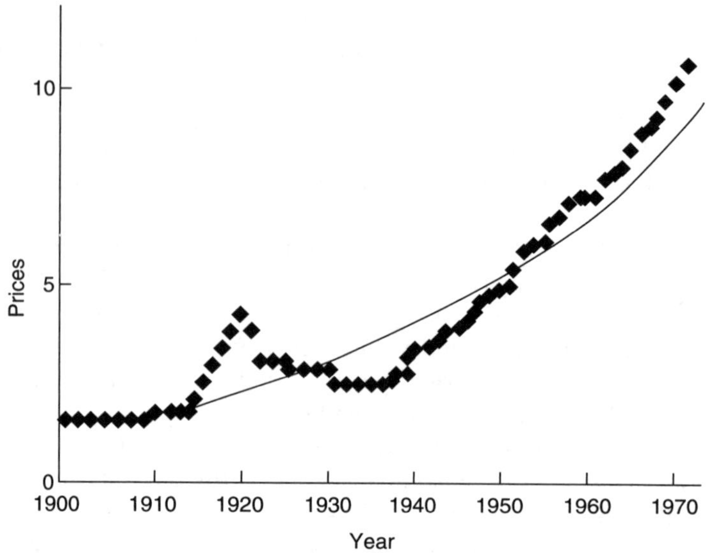

4.13 Index of prices in Great Britain (2000 = 100) 1900–1970. Average annual increase: 2.7%.

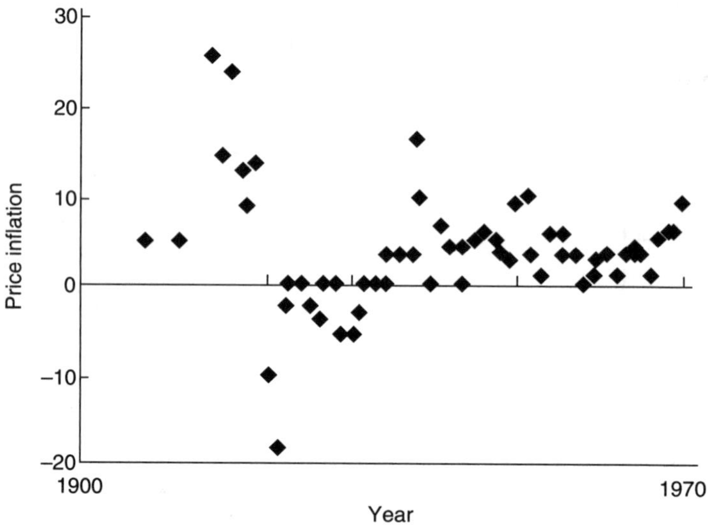

4.14 Annual percentage price inflation in Great Britain 1900–1970.

The linear phase is plotted in Fig. 4.15. The data points conform very closely to the best-fit straight line shown. In Fig. 4.12 this phase looks alarming but, in fact, linear price increases lead to a stable condition. Data conform to the equation

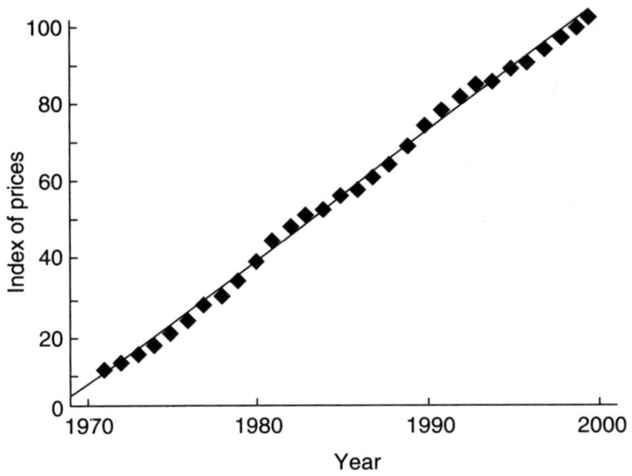

4.15 Index of prices in Great Britain 1970–2000.

$$P_t = at + b \qquad [4.1]$$

where P is the price index, t is time (in years) and a and b are constants.

Then, at any time t, the proportional annual increase in price is

$$\sigma = (P_{t+1} - P_t)/P_t \qquad [4.2]$$

$$= [(a(t+1)+b)-(at+b)]/(at+b) \qquad [4.3]$$

$$= \frac{1}{\left(t+\frac{b}{a}\right)} \qquad [4.4]$$

Thus, when the price index increases with time in a linear fashion, the inflation rate *decreases*. Figure 4.16 plots the annual inflation rate for Great Britain, shown as a percentage, between 1970 and 2000. By 1990 annual inflation had fallen to a low and more or less steady level. Figure 4.16 includes a plot of Equation [4.4], to which the data points conform reasonably well.

Prices and the inflation rate correspond with, and complement, economic growth data as indicators of human attitudes and behaviour. Inflation rate, for example, fell very sharply after the First World War and provided a good representation of the severity of the post-war depression. More surprising is the fact that they correlate with mortality rates. For men and women over the age of 45, mortality rates from all causes showed a

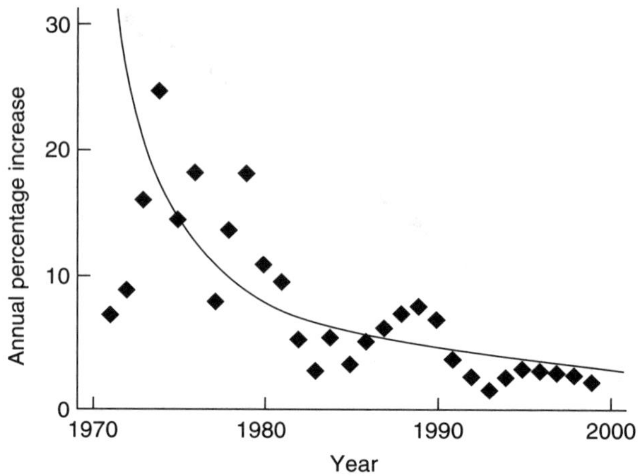

4.16 Annual percentage increase in prices in Great Britain 1970–2000.

consistent pattern during the twentieth century. For the first three-quarters of the period, they decreased exponentially in a very irregular fashion. Then, in the latter years, the fall became linear with very little scatter. For men, mortality rates due to accidents followed a similar course. Figure 4.17 is an example of the second phase: it shows all-cause and accident mortality rates for men in the age group 65 to 74 from 1970 to 2000.

Thus, prices and mortality rates followed a similar pattern during the twentieth century, except, of course, that they proceeded in the opposite sense: prices went up, but mortality rates went down.

Where such correlations have been observed for other activities, they have been ascribed to the fact that both records reflect human development as a whole, and such is considered to be the case here. Progress during the first part of the twentieth century was seriously affected by political instability and war in Europe. The reckless mood that resulted persisted for a while after the Second World War, and was eventually supplanted by more sober and cautious attitudes. Correspondingly, mortality rates for older persons declined, as did the rate of price inflation.

Younger age groups were not thus affected because their mortality rates had already fallen to a level beyond which only marginal improvements were possible. The date for this change was given earlier as 1970; however, all-cause mortality rates for older women started to decline in a linear fashion before this date, in the early 1960s, and accident mortality rates for some male age groups started to fall at the same time. The attitude change seems, therefore, to have taken place over a period of some years.

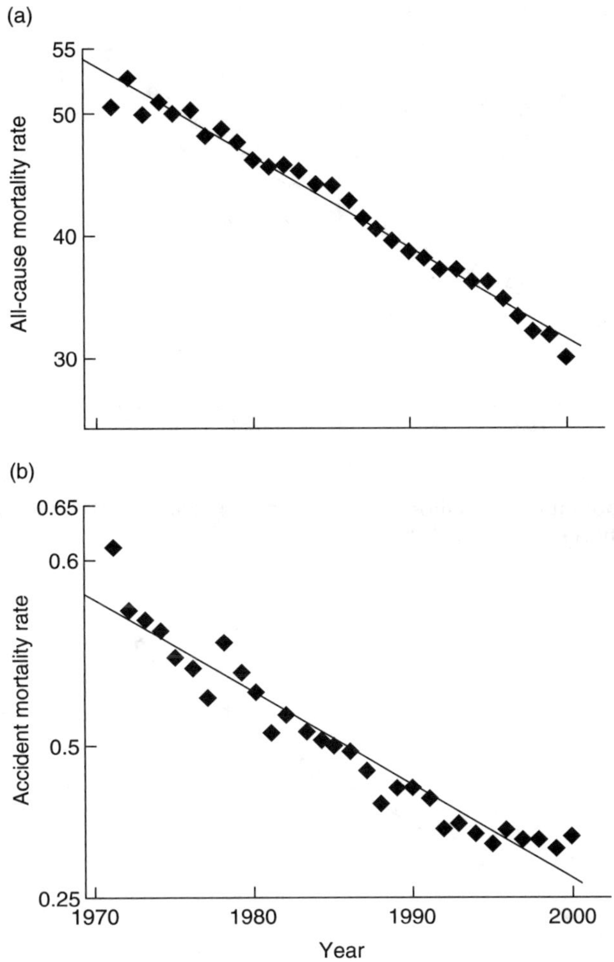

4.17 Mortality rates per 1000 population of the 65–74 age group in England and Wales 1970–2000 (a) from all causes (b) due to accidents.

4.7 Population trend in Britain 1801–2001

It has been customary in this book to use annual data in order to calculate trends. Population in Britain, however, is measured by means of a census taken every 10 years, and intermediate annual figures are calculated or interpolated. The first nationwide census in Britain was in 1841, but figures from parish and other local records are available for England and Wales from 1801. Therefore, 10-yearly figures from this date have been used here.

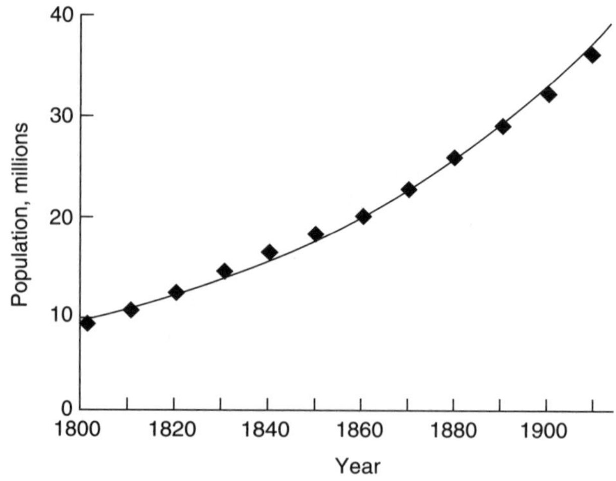

4.18 Population in millions of England and Wales, 1801–1911. Annual proportional increase: 1.3%.

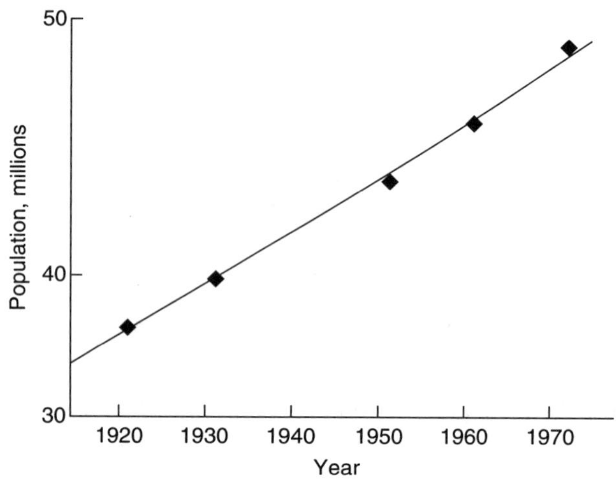

4.19 Population in millions of England and Wales, 1921–1971. Annual proportional increase: 0.5%.

Population growth in England and Wales has been exponential. The increase has occurred in three phases: from 1801 to 1911; from 1912 to 1971; and from 1971 to 2001. Data points and the relevant trend curves are shown in Figs. 4.18, 4.19 and 4.20. The proportional annual increase indicated by the trend curves decreases progressively, being 1.3% during the first phase, 0.5% during the second, and 0.22% during the third. In the first two phases the data points lie almost exactly on the trend curve. In the third phase the

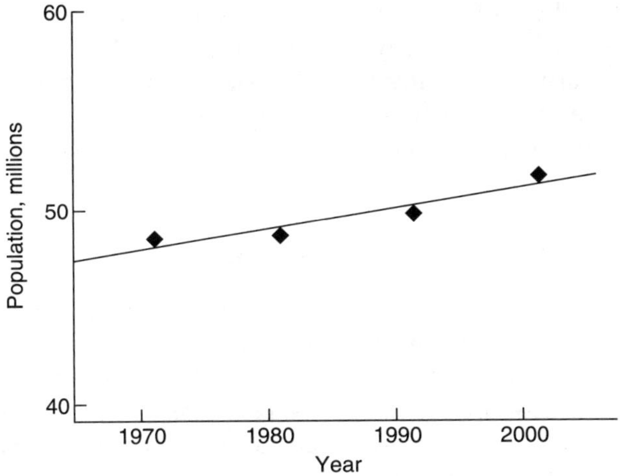

4.20 Population of England and Wales, 1971–2000. Annual proportional increase: 0.22%.

correlation is not quite so good, but would nevertheless rank statistically as a true correlation.

It will be evident that this last phase of lower population growth coincides with the period of reduced inflation and mortality rates which were enumerated in the previous section.

The record of population growth is significant in one other respect. A major conclusion of the present study is that human activity, as measured, for example, by economic growth rates, is regulated by the relevant population and (by implication) not by a superior authority. On the other hand, governments frequently claim that they control 'the economy', particularly when it is performing well. In the case of population growth; however, in Britain there is no regulating authority. The Census Office has a purely recording function. Nevertheless, as shown by Figs. 4.17 to 4.19, population growth in England and Wales is regulated with a high degree of precision. Therefore, the population itself must be responsible for regulation. Moreover, since this same population is not conscious of the mechanics of this process, or even that it exists, the regulation must be subconscious in character.

The first phase of population growth considered here encompassed the first half of the nineteenth century, when, by contemporary standards, mortality rates were extremely high, and the beginning of the twentieth century, when they had already fallen to a significant extent, particularly amongst infants and young children. Maintaining a constant proportional growth of population required a very precise adjustment of birth rate and family size. This task was accomplished without conscious effort or knowledge. Indeed, the only time that the public appeared to be aware of matters concerning population growth was in the early twentieth century, when the birth rate was falling (necessarily so, to match falling mortality rates) and some prophets began to foresee the extinction of the Anglo-Saxon race. But, as a rule, population growth in Britain arouses very little public interest.

4.8 Politics and economic growth

It was suggested earlier that, since economic growth is regulated by the population as a whole, the claims by politicians to be responsible for such growth must be questionable. Fortunately, the record for Great Britain for the second half of the twentieth century makes it possible to test the validity of such claims. The test to be applied is economic growth, as measured by the exponent of the trend curve for the relevant period.

The two main political parties, Labour and Conservative, have alternated in office since 1945 as follows:

Labour	1945–1951
Conservative	1951–1964
Labour	1964–1970
Conservative	1970–1974
Labour	1974–1979
Conservative	1979–1997

Of these, the first Labour period must be discounted because it includes the post-war recession. Also, the period of Edward Heath's government, 1970–1974, was too short to be statistically significant. The adjacent Labour terms have therefore been melded together. The result, with the calculated annual growth rate of the national output per head, is as follows:

Conservative	1951–1964:	2.257%
Labour	1964–1970, 1974–1979:	2.14%
Conservative	1979–1997:	2.146%

There is, in fact, no significant difference between these three results; the variation is well within the range that would be expected had the same political administration been in place for the whole period. In all cases the calculation was made using output data at constant prices, and the probability that the trend curve gave a true representation of the data was better than 0.999.

Thus, there was no significant difference between the economic growth rates under different political administration in Britain during the second half of the twentieth century. Such was the case in spite of the major economic reforms carried out whilst Margaret Thatcher was Prime Minister.

4.9 Regulating human behaviour

The evidence presented in the previous section is consistent with the idea that a democratic government is not capable of regulating economic growth to any significant extent, nor, would it seem, has such a government much influence on other modes of human behaviour. In the case of fatal accidents, however, there have been several attempts to do this.

The construction of oil refineries and petrochemical plants has, in the past, been notorious for a high incidence of fatal accidents, and several attempts have been made, in the USA and in Britain, to reduce the fatality rate by conscious endeavours. The technique relied, first and foremost, on obtaining the moral support of the workforce by discussion with trade unions and with the staff itself. Areas of special hazard and difficult access, or with special construction difficulties were identified and suitable action taken. There was regular inspection of trouble spots, and progress was reported to the workforce.

This type of activity, led in some cases by engineers and in others by psychologists, had a significant degree of success, although in some cases fatality rates appeared to reach an irreducibly low level. Also, fatality rates in the construction industry, in general, have begun to fall. A technique similar to that described above has been used in factories to reduce fatal accident rates, again with some degree of success.

Thus, it is possible to modify human behaviour by conscious effort. However, by their nature, such methods are only applicable to small groups of people. Large populations must be left to regulate themselves, which, as has been shown throughout this book, they do, as a rule, very well.

5

Analysing historical data: characteristics and methods

5.1 Quantitative history

The subject matter of this book does not fit comfortably into any contemporary academic discipline. It is, of course, based on the collection and analysis of historical records, but there are no kings and queens, no narrative, and no respectable historian would recognise its spotty diagrams as having anything to do with his or her craft. They do, however, tell a story. This has the virtue of being based on verifiable fact, and in many cases it follows an unexpected course.

The purpose of examining records of fatal accident rates is, in the first place, to determine how matters stand so far as safety is concerned. Are fatal accident rates increasing or decreasing? It emerges that, with a few well-defined exceptions (motorcycling for example), such rates are decreasing as fast as could reasonably be expected, and in Great Britain (which, in this matter, is typical of Western European countries) current procedures for the prevention of accidents are adequate. However, much else becomes evident. In particular, fatal accident rates and the rate of development generally are regulated collectively and subconsciously by the human population. Also, the historical records indicate from time to time changes in trend, associated with a change in human attitudes of which, consciously, we were, at the time, totally unaware. Thus, our activities may be consciously or subconsciously regulated; we live in two worlds, and both of these are essential to our well-being.

This is a very large conclusion at which to arrive, having proceeded from a very humble starting point. But the starting point is immaterial: the records for accident mortality, mortality from all causes, economic growth and population growth for Britain are all linked and show important common characteristics.

This, indeed, is the essence of the present study; that is, the assemblage and analysis of historical records of various activities as a means of observing human behaviour. This work has some common ground with history, psychology, philosophy and ergonomics, but it is not part of any of these subjects. For the present, the term 'quantitative history' will have to suffice. The potential field for research is, of course, very wide indeed: in this book only a tiny proportion of the data available worldwide has been studied.

5.2 Practical considerations

The instrument that appears to be best adapted to this work is the scientific graphing calculator, such as the Sharp EL-9900. This device has capabilities that are especially useful in statistical work. Firstly, it is designed to handle lists, and lists are the basic raw material thereof. These items may be handled in the same way as single algebraic variables. Thus, a list of annual deaths may be divided by a list of the relevant populations to provide a list of mortality rates. Secondly, it will plot one list against another and display the result on screen, whence the practised eye will be able to discern a trend. Thirdly, it will plot the relevant trend curve. These calculators may be linked to a computer to store or print out data or diagrams.

5.2.1 Units

The most generally useful unit of time is 1 year: this eliminates seasonal variations and at the same time provides adequate detail. Also annual data are needed for calculating variance. Five-year average figures are sometimes available, and are to be avoided. Exceptionally, longer intervals may be appropriate. In Britain, there is a census every 10 years, and thus 10-yearly figures were used in Chapter 4 for calculating population growth.

For true comparability, it is always desirable to use non-dimensional units. In statistical work this is rarely possible, but an example will be provided later. At least in the case of variance, the proportional value will normally be used here. Non-dimensional index numbers are often used in handling economic data. Otherwise, calculated units have been expressed so as to avoid unwieldy numbers.

5.2.2 Types of data and their analysis

Historical records exist for a very wide variety of human activities. Those of primary interest here include annual deaths due to accidents nationwide, and annual fatality numbers associated with the various modes of transport and in different industries. Related data are mortality rates from all causes, together with economic indicators, including growth rates, national productivity and price inflation. Population numbers are required for calculating mortality rates, but are also of interest in their own right. Sources used in this book are listed in the Appendix.

Suppose that the lists of two finite variables, $L1$ and $L2$, have been made, and it is required to find the relationship between these two and plot the relevant trend curve. The procedure is as follows:

(1) Select the independent quantity as the x-variable.
(2) Take the logarithms of both lists.
(3) In a plot of $\log L1$ and $\log L2$, find the straight line such that the sum of the squares of the vertical displacements of data points from this line is a minimum.
(4) Take antilogarithms and replot.

If time is one of the variables, this is then the independent one, $L1$, and is left unchanged. The plot is then between $L1$ and $\log L2$. Otherwise, the procedure is the same.

Provided that the expected relationship between the two sets of variables (e.g. $y = ax + b$, a straight line) is specified, the calculator will carry out this procedure using the two lists $L1$ and $L2$. It will also display the correlation coefficient r. This is a figure that indicates whether or not the correlation is accidental or true. It varies numerically from 0 to 1; zero indicates no correlation, and 1 that all data points lie precisely on the trend curve. The correlation coefficients for the diagrams presented in Chapters 1 to 4 are nearly all greater than 0.9; that for population growth during the nineteenth century being 0.995. There is therefore no reason to doubt their validity.

5.3 Quantifying a trend

It has been shown in earlier chapters that, subject to perturbations by major events such as the two World Wars, the various measures of human activities vary in a well-regulated manner with time, and consequently may be represented by formal mathematical relationships, which may be capable of generating a *trend curve*. They may also be subject to sudden changes of direction, due to unstable conditions. And the variation of data relative to the trend curve may also occur in a regular fashion. The latter two items will be considered later under the headings 'Instabilities' and 'Variance'.

Four types of mathematical relationship may be of use: linear, hyperbolic, exponential and sinusoidal.

The linear trend has been encountered in all the records considered in this book. It is represented by:

$$R = ax + b \qquad [5.1]$$

where R is the rate of loss or gain, x is the independent variable, whilst a and b are constants.

The hyperbolic form is:

$$R = \frac{a}{x^b} \qquad [5.2]$$

where the symbols have the same meaning as in Equation [5.1].

The hyperbolic relationships may only be used when x is a finite quantity; an example is the plot of road fatality rates against national productivity in Chapter 1. It cannot be employed when the independent variable is time, because there is no finite measure of time.

The exponential relationship is:

$$R = ae^{bx} \qquad [5.3]$$

with symbols as before. This form is applicable when x represents time. When b is positive, it indicates an increase, as in population growth; when it is negative, there is a fall, as with the reduction of accident mortality over a period of time. The quantity 'b' is not necessarily constant, but may vary with time either continuously or in steps. In all the trend curves plotted in previous chapters, however, b has been assumed to be constant.

Sinusoidal variation may be expressed as:

$$R_s = a \sin\left(\frac{2\pi x}{\lambda}\right) \qquad [5.4]$$

where λ is the wavelength (in time) of the displacement. Sinusoidal variation may occur during economic growth, as shown in Figs 4.3 and 4.5. Here, it is combined with exponential increase, such that Equation [5.3] must be multiplied by R_s.

5.4 The exponential case

Exponential change is the most common trend to be found in the historical records examined here. The national output per head of Great Britain and its population increase exponentially whilst, for the most part, fatality rates in industry and in the various modes of transport decrease in a similar manner.

A ruling characteristic of exponential change is that the proportional gradient is constant; that is to say, that for the corresponding trend curve, the gradient at any point, divided by the value of the ordinate at the same point, remains the same regardless of position. Thus, for a system where the rate R is changing exponentially with time t,

$$\frac{1}{R}\frac{dR}{dt} = b \qquad [5.5]$$

separating variables and integrating gives:

$$\ln R = bt + \text{constant} \qquad [5.6]$$

or

$$R = ae^{bt} \qquad [5.7]$$

since, in equation [5.6] $\ln R$ is the logarithm of R to base e.

When data rise with time, as in the case of economic growth, the constant b is positive, whilst in a falling trend it is negative.

The numerical value of b obtained using the analytical method outlined earlier in this chapter is, for historical records considered here, typically between 0.01 and 0.06. The figure $100 \times b$ has been used in earlier chapters to indicate the percentage annual increase or decrease of, for example, fatality rates. This is not strictly correct. The annual exponential change is:

$$\frac{(R_{t+1} - R_t)}{R_t} = \frac{(ae^{b(t+1)} - ae^{bt})}{ae^{bt}} = e^b - 1 \qquad [5.8]$$

Suppose $b = 0.05$, then $e^b - 1 = 0.05127\ldots$

The inaccuracy is of no consequence in expressing a percentage annual change, but needs to be considered when making calculations.

Thus there are two ways to obtain a value of the parameter b. The first is to calculate the trend curve. This is the standard route and gives a pictorial image of the trend; it also permits an estimate of the variance, as will be seen later. The other method is to calculate the proportional fall for each year and take the average. Data obtained in this way show a great deal of scatter but, by compensation, they may indicate a variation of b with time.

Finally, if the average proportional annual change is $\bar{x}$, then $b = \ln(1 + \bar{x})$.

Now it is entirely reasonable to suppose that, where the value of b increases, then human behaviour in the activity concerned is becoming more reckless, whilst if it is decreasing then caution has prevailed. Thus, it was shown earlier that, for the 10-year period after the use of seat belts was made compulsory in Britain, the slope of the trend curve for fatality rates decreased as compared with the previous 10-year period, with a corresponding increase in the value of b. At the same time, there was an increase in the rate of pedestrian deaths, confirming that motorcar drivers were operating more recklessly.

Quantitatively, the effect of the seat belt law was not very considerable. However, it was found in Chapters 3 and 4 that various records indicated a general change to more cautious behaviour in Great Britain after 1970. Accordingly, Figure 5.1 is a plot of the annual proportional change in the fatality rate due to road accidents in Britain for 1934 to 2000. The trend lines for 1934–1970 and 1970–2000 have been calculated separately and are shown. The pre-1970 period does indeed conform to expectations: there is an increase in the value of b, whilst after 1970 it remains almost constant.

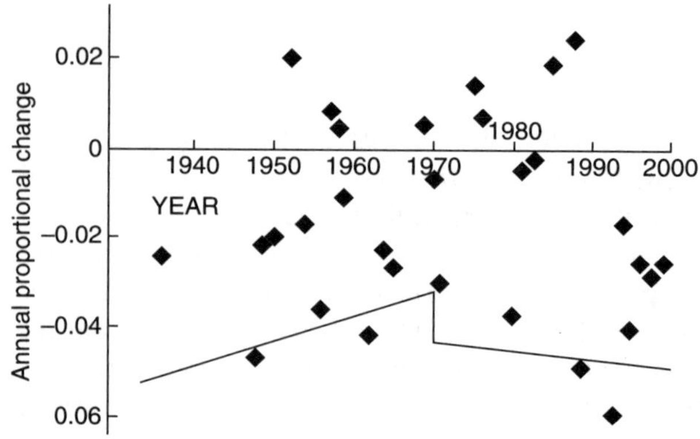

5.1 Annual proportional change of fatality rate due to accidents on British roads, 1934–1970 and 1970–2000. Because of the wide scatter some data points have been omitted from this figure and from Fig. 5.2. All data were taken into account in calculating the trend lines, however.

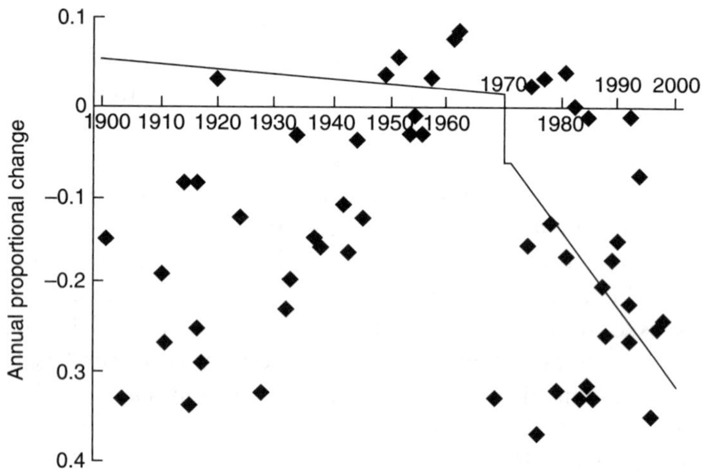

5.2 Annual proportional change of male all-cause mortality rate of England and Wales 1901–1970 and 1970–2000. The diagram shows only a limited range of data points; these vary from −0.11 to +0.12. All data points were taken into account when calculating the trend lines.

A similar exercise has been performed with all-cause mortality rates in England and Wales for the male 65–74 age group. In this instance it was known from a straightforward plot of mortality rates that a sharp linear drop occurred after 1970 or thereabouts. Figure 5.2 demonstrates that the annual proportional change plot tells a similar story. Once again, however, the scatter of data points is uncomfortably wide.

The value of b obtained by taking an average of annual values differs slightly from that obtained from trend curve calculations. Thus, in the case of road accident fatality rates in Britain from 1934 to 2000, excluding the war years, b from the trend curve is –0.0456. The average of the annual proportional change is –0.0506, so the corresponding value of b is $\ln(1 - 0.0506) = -0.0519$. Bearing in mind the large year-to-year scatter of the annual proportional change values, this is as good an agreement as could be expected. In any event, the trend curve figure is preferred.

Most of the historical numerical records of human activities are best represented by an exponential trend curve. Both economic growth and population growth are exponential; the data points for population growth in England and Wales, plotted at 10-year intervals, fall almost precisely on the relevant trend curve. Fatality rates due to accidents are a great deal less precise, but in the case of most industries and modes of transport follow a falling exponential trend which, in the case of road accidents, is very well ordered. All-cause mortality rates fell during the twentieth century, and for children and young adults may reasonably be represented by an exponential curve. For those over the age of 45, matters are more complicated, and will be considered shortly.

Data sets that follow a linear course fall into one of two categories. In the first, the data are widely scattered, and the gradient of the trend line relatively low; the second type has a narrow scatter band and a relatively steep slope.

Figure 5.3 provides good examples of these two modes. It is a plot of all-cause and accident mortalities for the male 65–74 age group in England and Wales between 1901 and 2000. The pattern outlined by the data points is the same in both cases: prior to 1970, there was considerable scatter and a slow downward drift; after this date, the scatter was small and the slope steep. Quantitatively, the relative standard deviation is, before 1970 for all-cause mortality, 0.058 and, for accidents 0.18, post-1970 the figures are, respectively, 0.017 and 0.033.

A similar pattern was observed in the case of all-cause mortality rates for children and young adults in the nineteenth century before and after 1870; also for price inflation in the twentieth century, although in this case the trend was, of course, upwards.

The linear trend line is usually represented as

$$R = at + b \qquad [5.9]$$

where R represents a rate, t is time and a and b are constants, a being the slope.

When the trend curve equation is determined using the method outlined earlier in this chapter and the criterion that the sum of the squares of displacement of data points from the curve is a minimum, then it is required that, in the case of a linear trend, the line should pass through the point $\bar{t}$,

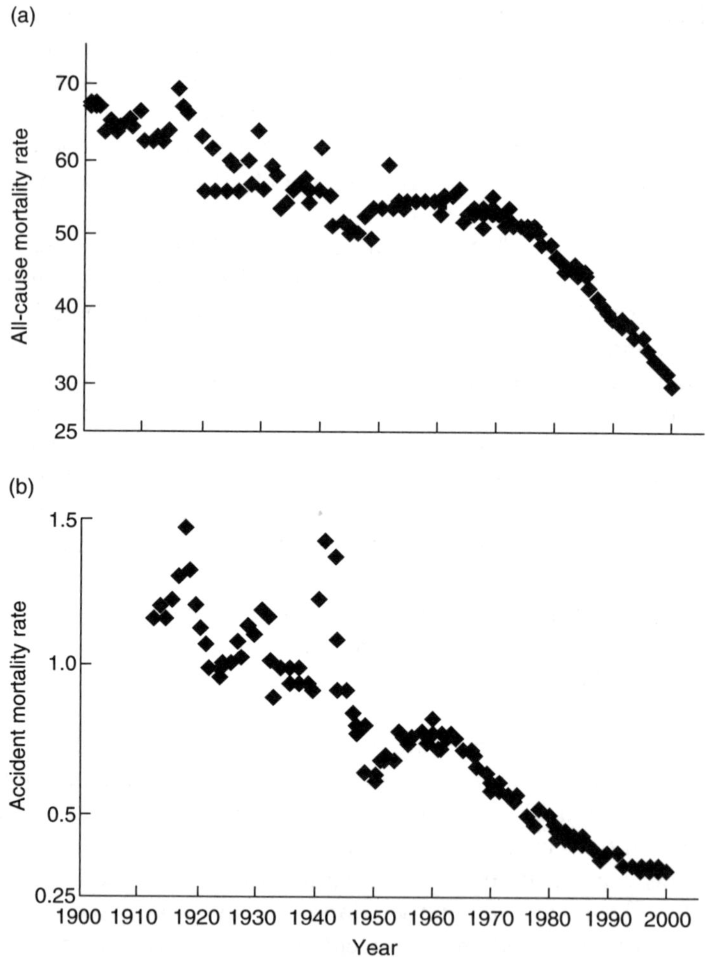

5.3 Mortality rate per 1000 population in England and Wales for the 65–74 age group 1901–2000 (a) from all causes (b) due to accidents.

$\bar{R}$, where these are averages of the t and R ordinates, respectively. Thus, $b = \bar{R} - a\bar{t}$ and

$$R - \bar{R} = a(t - \bar{t}) \qquad [5.10]$$

This is a more elegant form and is used in deriving the linear trend equation. Equation [5.9] is, however, more generally applicable.

A notable case of rising linear trend is that concerning prices in Britain between 1970 and 2000. For a rising trend the gradient is positive, so that the inflation rate $\Delta R/R$ followed a decreasing, hyperbolic course, as shown in Fig. 4.15.

A downward linear trend is observed in sets of all-cause and accident mortality data for age groups 45–54 and higher, and most frequently with those for the period 1970–2000. As with all historical data related to human activities, there are irregularities. In some instances, particularly in the case of females, the downturn began as early as 1950; in others, the apparently linear trend is better represented by an exponential trend curve, but for the most part the trend is linear, with little scatter.

5.5 The hyperbolic case

It was observed that a hyperbolic trend may be appropriate when the independent variable is finite. it is also a necessary relationship when both quantities vary exponentially with time: for example, national output per head, which will be regarded here as the independent variable, R_x, and the fatality rate due to road accidents, designated R_y. The exponential relationships are:

$$R_x = ae^{bt} \text{ and } R_y = ce^{dt} \qquad [5.11]$$

and therefore, for any time t

$$t = \frac{1}{b}\ln\frac{R_n}{a} = \frac{1}{a}\ln\frac{R_y}{c} \qquad [5.12]$$

so that $(R_x/a)^{1/b} = (R_y/c)^{1/a}$

or $R_y = mR_n^{d/b}$

where

$$m = \frac{c}{a^{d/b}} \qquad [5.13]$$

In Great Britain, b is approximately 6.02 and d is about –0.045, so that $d/b \simeq -0.0075$.

Figure 5.4 is a plot of the relevant data points for Great Britain between 1934 and 2000, excluding those for the war years. The trend curve coincides with the data point plot except at the start, prior to 1947.

5.6 The sinusoidal case

In Chapter 4 it was observed that plots of national output per head for Great Britain in the second half of the nineteenth and twentieth centuries followed a fluctuating course relative to the trend curve, and that this course was roughly sinusoidal in form. Overall, economic growth was exponential, so the data could be represented by the expression

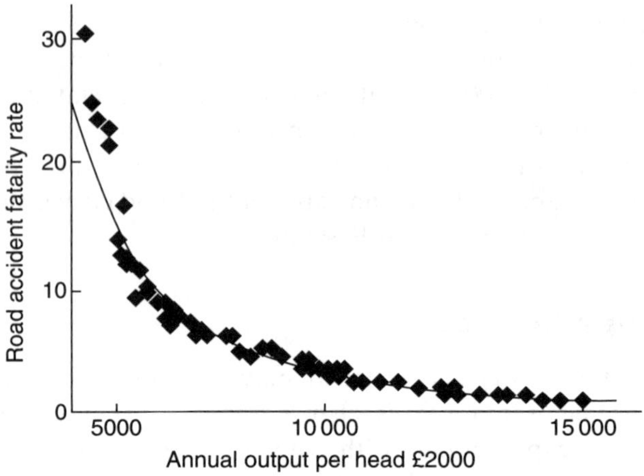

5.4 Hyperbolic relationship between fatality rate due to road accidents and per capita gross domestic product (PCGDP) in Great Britain 1934–2000, excluding the war years. PCGDP is expressed in pounds sterling for the year 2000 and annual road deaths are per 10 000 vehicles. The trend curve is $y = 516/x^{2.2}$.

$$R = \left[f(t)\sin\left(\frac{2\pi t}{\lambda}\right) \times ae^{bt} \right] \quad [5.14]$$

In this expression $f(t)$ represents the amplitude and λ the wavelength (inverse of frequency) of the perturbation. It was also found that the amplitude of the variation increased with time up to a point where there was a sudden collapse, in 1891 and 1989, respectively.

Suppose that the national output per head at any date is R_i and the corresponding trend curve is R_t, then the proportional deviation of the data point is $(R_i - R_t)/R_t = P$. Values of P may be plotted independently of the trend curve, and they are given by a sinusoidal curve. Assuming that the amplitude of perturbations increases in a linear fashion with time, the P data may be represented by

$$P = C(t - t_0)\sin\left(\frac{2\pi(t - t_0)}{\lambda}\right) \quad [5.15]$$

In this expression t_0 is the start date and t_1 moves the curve laterally to provide a good fit to the data.

Figure 5.5 is a plot of the proportional deviations from the trend curve for the period 1855 to 1899. For the sinusoidal curve, with time listed 55, 56, 57 . . . 99, $t_0 = 55$ and $t_1 = 50$. Deviations are shown as a percentage of the trend curve value. There are three 10-year cycles of increasing amplitude, whilst the fourth curve is interrupted in 1891 by a catastrophic fall.

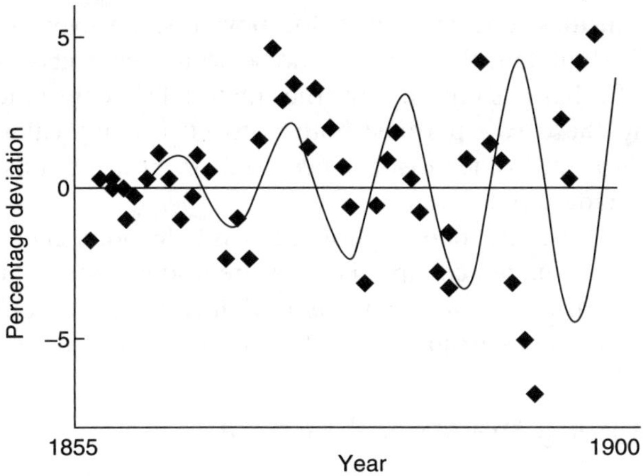

5.5 Percentage deviation of data points from trend curve for national output per head in Great Britain 1855–1899, with sinusoidal model.

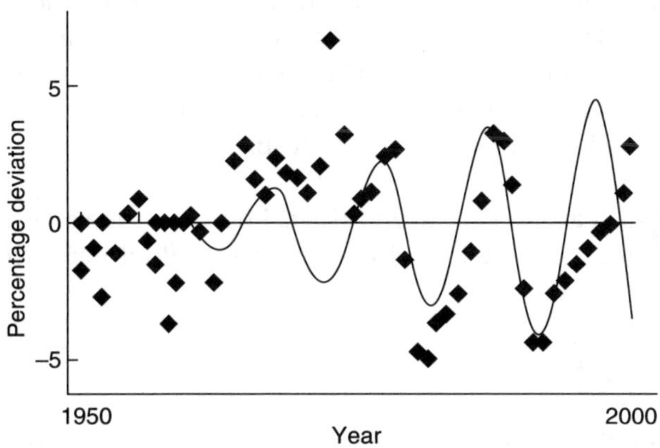

5.6 Percentage deviation of data points from trend curve for national output per head in Great Britain 1950–2000.

This pattern of events is analogous to the motion of a pendulum, which receives an impulse as it passes the bottom dead centre. The swings become progressively wider until eventually it goes over the top. Similarly, the human behaviour represented by Fig. 5.5 is progressively more reckless until it reaches an unacceptable level and there is a collapse.

Figure 5.6 is a similar plot for the period 1950–2000. The sinusoidal model superimposed is the same as that for 1885–1899, with the sole exception that $t_1 = 45$. In this instance the curve fits better in the latter part of the period but overall agreement is much the same. The final collapse, however, was much less severe in this case. For both periods the downswings reflect economic recessions.

The idea that history repeats itself is not new; it is, however, somewhat disturbing that it should, in this instance, do so with such precision. There was, of course, a basic similarity in the material circumstances that pertained during these two periods: both enjoyed relative calm after a half-century of war and other disturbances, and in both periods science and technology made rapid advances.

However this may be, the tendency for reckless behaviour to build up to a peak followed by a sudden collapse is a feature also of some fatality rate records, as noted earlier. Such behaviour is characteristic of young men, who may indeed provide a substantial contribution to those ups and downs.

5.7 Quantifying the spread of data

Objects that occur naturally and in quantity are variable in their measurable quantities such as size and weight, and the extent and character of such variation is an essential characteristic of a particular batch or sample. Consider, for example, the birth weight of babies born during one year in a particular country. There is an average or mean weight of this group, and the actual weight of babies tends to cluster around this mean; that is to say, birth weights close to the average are greatest in numbers, and numbers become progressively fewer the farther the birth weight varies from the mean.

The extent of such a spread of properties is known as the variance, which is defined as the mean of squares of the difference of all items from their average:

$$\mathrm{VAR} = \frac{1}{n}\sum (x_i - \bar{x})^2 \qquad [5.16]$$

where n is the number of items, x_i is the property of any item, and $\bar{x}$ is the average property.

The square root of the variance is known as the standard deviation, designated by the lower case Greek letter sigma, σ. The standard deviation is a measure of the spread of data, and, in modified form, was used in Chapter 2 to define the boundaries of a set of time-dependent quantities.

These quantities were fatality and loss rates due to accidents, and it is found that the rules which apply to physical objects such as the size of hens' eggs or the weight of rice grains also apply to more abstract measurements, such as fatality rates. However, there are two features of such measurements that need to be kept in mind.

The first point is that, in most instances, an individual figure is, itself, an average. Consider, for example, accident mortality rates for males as depicted in Fig. 3.5. From the data from which this figure was developed, it could be concluded that the level of acceptable risk for males was such-and-such. However, males vary in their nature from very reckless to very cautious, and there is no way in which this variation can be quantified. Thus, the variability of accident mortality data is the variability of averages, and not that of individual human beings.

Secondly, the systems considered here always have two variables, and the variation of data is with respect to a trend curve, not to an average. Also, in most cases the trend is a diminishing one, and it is found empirically that the width of scatter bands falls in proportion to this trend. Thus the significant variable is the proportional deviation from the trend curve. Suppose that the ordinate of any data point is R_i, and the corresponding value of the trend curve (for the year t_i) is Rt_i, then

$$[\mathrm{VAR}]_r = \frac{1}{n}\sum\frac{(R_i - Rt_i)^2}{Rt_i^2} \qquad [5.17]$$

where $Rt_i^2 = ae^{bti}$

$[\mathrm{VAR}]_r$ is the relative variance, and its square root is the relative standard deviation σ_r. Both these quantities are non-dimensional and are therefore comparable, regardless of the nature of the activity they represent or the absolute value of the loss rate. There are a number of instances where a plot of data against time is best represented by a straight line. These include the rising trend of road accident fatality rates in Britain between 1926 and 1934, and the falling trend of accident and all-cause mortality rates in England and Wales between 1870 and 1899 and between 1970 and 2000. In these plots the spread of data points relative to the trend line is more or less constant, and the relative variance is:

$$[\mathrm{VAR}]_r = \frac{1}{n}\sum\frac{(R_i - Rt_i)^2}{\bar{R}_i^2} \qquad [5.18]$$

where symbols are as before and $\bar{R}_i$ is the average of rates.

The standard deviation is a more generally useful quantity than the variance. It gives a realistic comparison for the degree of scatter in plots of different periods or different activities.

5.8 Frequency distribution

Suppose that a set of data is arranged in accordance with their deviation from the average or, as is normal here, in accordance with their proportional deviation from the trend curve, the frequency f at any particular deviation is the proportion of data that exists at this point. Thus, if the total number of data is n, and deviations are plotted on the x-axis as proportions of the total, an approximation to the frequency is:

$$f = \frac{1}{n}\frac{\Delta n}{\Delta x}$$

and where f becomes a continuous function:

$$f = \frac{1}{n}\frac{dn}{dx} \qquad [5.19]$$

In the case of most natural phenomena, and for such data as accident mortality rates, the frequency is a maximum when the deviation is zero; that is, when the measured quantity is equal to the average or lies exactly on the trend curve. If the proportional deviation is $x = (R_i - R_{ti})/R_{ti}$, then a plot of f against x will produce a curve that will peak at $x = 0$ and diminish for increasing and decreasing values of x. Also, if the scatter of data is small, the peak will be relatively narrow and high, whilst with a wide scatter band, the frequency plot will be relatively flat. In principle, such frequency plots extend from minus infinity to plus infinity.

The mathematician Gauss found that the frequency of astronomical errors made by students could be represented by the expression:

$$f = \frac{1}{\sqrt{\pi}} e^{-x^2} \qquad [5.20]$$

The factor $\frac{1}{\sqrt{\pi}}$ arises because $\int_{-\infty}^{\infty} e^{-x^2} dx = \sqrt{\pi}$ and $\int_{-\infty}^{\infty} f = 1$. In order to determine whether or not the historic data examined here conform to this (Gaussian) distribution, put $x = (R_i - R_{ti})/a$. Now, suppose that R_i is a continuous variable, the variance is $[\text{VAR}] = \sigma^2 = \int_{-\infty}^{\infty} (R_i - R_{Ti})^2 dn$

$$= \int_{-\infty}^{\infty} a^2 x^2 \frac{1}{\sqrt{\pi}} e^{-x^2} dx$$

And since

$$\int_{-\infty}^{\infty} x^2 e^{-x^2} dx = \frac{\sqrt{\pi}}{4}$$

$$\sigma^2 = \frac{a^2}{2}$$

So

$$x = \frac{(R_i - R_{T_i})}{\sqrt{2}\sigma}$$

A similar process leads to

$$x = \frac{\left(\frac{R_i}{R_{T_i}} - 1\right)}{\sqrt{2}\sigma_r}$$

5.9 The 2σ boundaries

It will be evident that

$$\frac{1}{\sqrt{\pi}}\int_{-x}^{x} e^{-x^2}\,dx = \frac{2}{\sqrt{\pi}}\int_{0}^{x} e^{-x^2}\,dx$$

This quantity is known as the *error function*, because of its association with the errors of Professor Gauss's students. It is also significant in relation to human error generally, as will be seen below. The error function is tabulated or it may be calculated from the series:

$$\operatorname{erf} x = \frac{2}{\sqrt{\pi}}\sum_{n=0}^{\infty}\frac{(-1)^n x^{2n+1}}{(2n+1)n!} \qquad [5.21]$$

Suppose that the proportional displacement is set at $2\sigma_r$, then $x = \sqrt{2}$ and $\operatorname{erf} x = 0.95449\ldots$ This means that, if its boundaries are set at a proportional distance of $2\sigma_r$ from the trend curve, and the frequency distribution is Gaussian, about 95% of data points will be enclosed within these boundaries. If the trend curve is $R = ae^{bt}$, then the boundaries are $(1 + 2\sigma_r)ae^{bt}$ and $(1 - 2\sigma_r)ae^{bt}$.

Almost all the data sets examined here conform to the 95% limit, although this does not, of course, confirm that their frequency distribution is Gaussian.

5.10 Plotting the distribution function

In order to calculate individual values of the frequency of any set of data, it is necessary to return to an earlier definition:

$$f = \frac{\Delta n}{n\Delta x} \qquad [5.22]$$

The procedure is as follows:

(1) Calculate the relative standard deviation for the data

$$\sigma_r^{\,2} = \frac{1}{n}\sum\frac{R_i - R_{T_i}}{R_{T_i}}$$

(2) Calculate values of x for each data point

$$x = \frac{\left(\dfrac{R_i}{R_{T_i}} - 1\right)}{\sqrt{2}\sigma}$$

(3) Arrange the list of x values in numerical order

(4) Select a range of Δx, say 0.5, and count the number of x values within successive ranges, –2.5 to –2, –2 to –1.5, etc.

(5) Calculate the frequency $f = \Delta n / n\Delta x$ for each interval of x.
(6) Plot the f values at the midpoint of each x range: –2.25, –1.75, etc.

This procedure has been followed for data concerned with three different activities: fatality rates due to accidents on British roads from 1950 to 2000, the national output per head in Great Britain for the period 1855 to 1899, and the annual percentage loss of steam and motor ships from the world's fleet from 1900 to 2000, other than the war periods. The results are plotted in Figs. 5.7, 5.8 and 5.9, respectively. In these diagrams the solid line

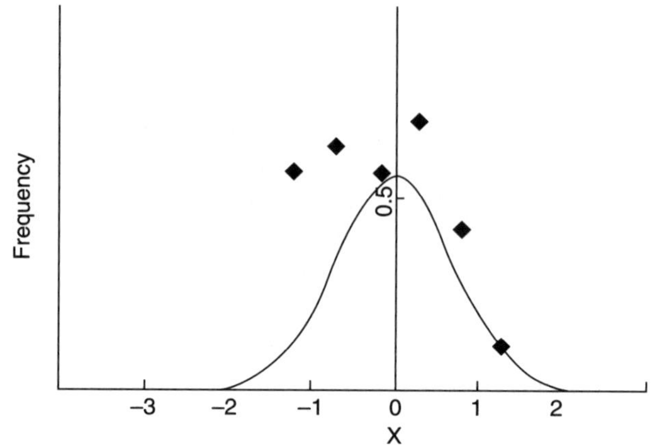

5.7 Frequency distribution of deviations from trend curve for fatality rate in road accidents in Britain 1950–2000 compared with Gaussian distribution (solid curve).

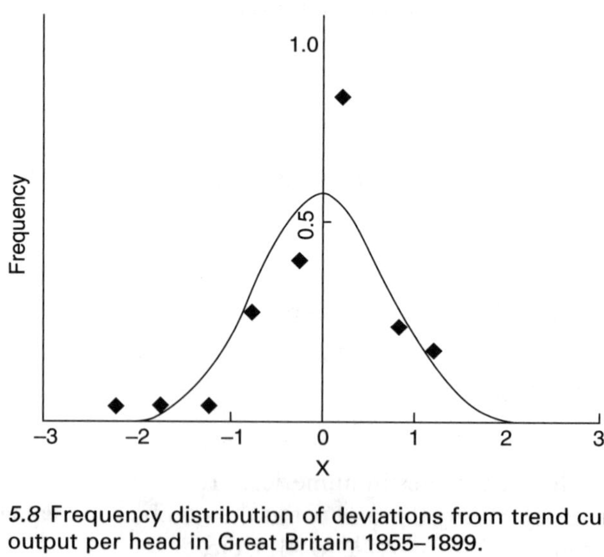

5.8 Frequency distribution of deviations from trend curve for national output per head in Great Britain 1855–1899.

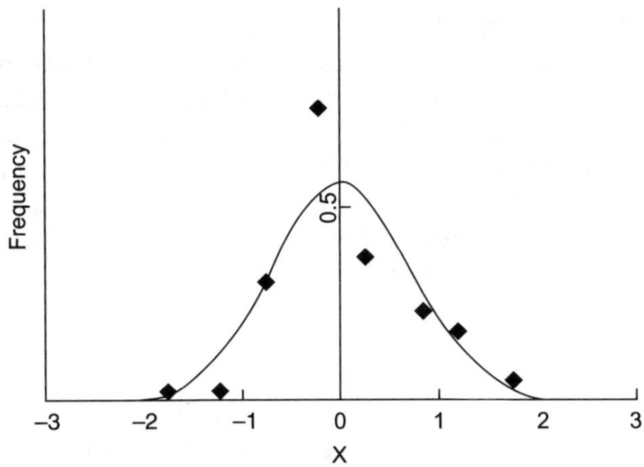

5.9 Frequency distribution of deviations from trend curve of percentage loss of steam and motor ships from the world's commercial fleet 1900–2000, excluding the two World War periods.

represents the expression $f = \frac{l}{\sqrt{\pi}} e^{-x^2}$ and the data points are set at intervals of 0.5. Figures 5.7 and 5.9 relate to exponentially falling rates, but Fig. 5.8 is for a rising trend. In general, agreement with the Gaussian model is good, and the same applies to most of the data sets that have been examined previously. This confirmation is important because, as demonstrated in this section, much of the mathematical framework that is assumed in the present analysis is based on Gaussian distribution.

5.11 The neutral condition

Suppose that $\sigma = 1/\sqrt{2}$, then $x = (R_i - R_{Ti})/R_{Ti}$ or $(R_i/R_{Ti} - 1)$, and a plot of the frequency distribution of this quantity, instead of being relatively peaked or flat, should conform to the bell-shaped curve shown in Figs. 5.7 to 5.9. By the same token: if σ is less than $1/\sqrt{2}$ (say, less than 0.707) the appropriate plot will be relatively peaked, and if it is greater, the plot will be relatively flat.

In all the data sets examined here, the value of the relative standard deviation is less than 0.707. In all the activities so represented, there is a positive human motivation; in the case of accident mortality, the will to preserve life, and in the case of economic growth, the desire for self-betterment. The relative standard deviation, therefore, may be more than a bleak statistical quantity; it can be an indicator of human (or other animal) motivation.

To reinforce this view, consider the case of a system in which the interactions are purely physical: a volume of gas in thermal equilibrium and at rest relative to its environment. The molecules thereof are exceedingly small and numerous, and they are in a state of constant motion. The components of velocity in a particular direction, v_z for example, range from zero to high positive and negative values, and since the gas is at rest, their average velocity component is zero. It has been shown that the frequency distribution of velocity components of such gas molecules is:

$$f = \frac{1}{\sqrt{\pi}} e^{-v^2/v_0^2}$$

where v is any velocity component and v_0 is constant and equal to the thermal velocity. Thus for such a purely physical system, $x = v/v_0$ and therefore $\sigma = 1/\sqrt{2}$ Thus, where human motivation is lacking, the frequency distribution is neither peaked nor flat: it is neutral.

Thus, it would appear that the condition where the relative standard deviation σ_r is equal to $1/\sqrt{2}$ constitutes a borderline between the data sets representing living and non-living matter. There are, however, practical considerations to be borne in mind. In the case of fatality rates due to transport, for example, the scatter of data is affected by the size of the vehicle. The two World Wars caused substantial distortions of accident and all-cause mortality data. Even when such distortions are included, though, the values of σ_r for the activities considered in this and previous chapters fall below the critical figure, and in many instances, very far below.

6
Some outstanding questions

6.1 Introduction

The facts presented in previous chapters of this book pose a series of awkward questions. It has been established that, for most industries and forms of transport, fatality rates due to accidents fall with the passage of time. This being so, what purpose is there in writing codes, standards and specifications that are designed with that end in mind? Mortality rates fall in a similar manner independently of the effectiveness of medical treatment, so what function do doctors and health services perform? And economic growth (in Britain) continues steadily regardless of political complexion of the government, so how effective is a government in regulating national affairs?

These are very large questions, but before attempting to answer them it is necessary to give some thought to a subject that is common to all; namely, subconscious learning and the subconscious regulation of human activities.

It is not easy to accept the view that such important matters as safety, longevity and economic growth should be regulated subconsciously by ordinary people, acting collectively. It is widely believed that human affairs are guided by the exercise of conscious, rational thought, and that they are directed by a higher authority: God, the King, a dictator or, at a pinch, a prime minister. On the other hand, two of our most vital assets, the ability to communicate by talking and that of walking upright, are self-evidently the result of subconscious learning. And, the evidence for subconscious regulation presented in earlier chapters of this book is very positive indeed.

Ever since stock markets first appeared in Western Europe, they have been plagued by instability in the price of shares, and from time to time a wholesale collapse occurs; most notoriously, the Wall Street crash of 1929. Such events are sometimes ascribed to the sin of avarice, or greed, or to some such unsavoury human characteristic. However, the record of productive activity that occurred during the second halves of the nineteenth and twentieth centuries also showed alternating periods of boom and slump. The term used to characterise behaviour during the boom phase was, in this instance 'recklessness'. To cast the net still wider: fatality rates due to losses of offshore mobile craft rose to a peak in the late twentieth century and then fell suddenly to a low point.

The common feature of these various events is the sudden change (of activity, or of fatality or loss rate) from a high to a low level. Such changes are judged to be due to a change of attitude by those concerned. Characteristically, there is no record at the conscious level (in newspaper or narrative history, for example) of such changes, which must therefore be classed as subconscious.

The fact that boom-and-bust is a feature of such varied activities, suggests that it is linked to a basic, identifiable human characteristic. The most likely candidate is the young adult male for whom the acceptable level of risk is high. Thus, young men take the lead during the boom phase, then, when the actual rise reaches an unacceptable level, suddenly switch their attitude to one of caution. So there is an abrupt fall in loss or economic growth rate; after which the cycle restarts. At no stage do the participants feel avaricious or greedy, they are just doing their job, albeit, perhaps, over-zealously.

6.2 Fatal accidents

This chapter began with a question: since accident mortality rates are falling in a regulated way, what purpose is served in writing engineering codes of practice that are aimed at promoting safety?

Firstly, engineering codes are not written solely, or even primarily, to promote safety. Lloyd's Register of Shipping was set up as the inspection arm of Lloyd's Insurance: it classifies ships in accordance with the seaworthiness of the hull and the quality of the fittings: given a good report, a ship was insurable. Later, Lloyd's rules for ship construction evolved, and these (much modified) exist today as a widely accepted standard. The primary motive here was to regulate financial risk. It is very probable that this process helped to improve standards of ship construction and thus reduce the mortality rate or seaman, but this is not certain and it was not the primary objective.

Likewise, in the early twentieth century, a group of British insurance companies set up the 'Associated Offices Technical Committee' to write rules for the construction of boilers and pressure vessels. Here, again, the primary aim was to provide justification for insurance cover. Regardless of insurability, however, construction to an accepted code provides a purchaser with an assurance of adequate quality.

Construction codes also have an educational function. Being written (hopefully) by experts who are aware of the latest technology and design theory, they should provide sound contemporary guidance to the relevant industry and its designers.

Failures in service of pressure vessels and boilers constructed according to code requirements occur from time to time in oil refineries and petrochemical plant: these were described in Chapter 2 and will be discussed later in this chapter. Otherwise, failures of major public works are rare. For the most part, structures are not exposed to severe conditions, but this caveat does not apply in the case of earthquakes. The Los Angeles building code is periodically given a very thorough destructive test, which, to date, the city has survived very well. The code *was* written with safety as the price incentive. It was started following an earthquake which occurred early in the morning and caused a school building to collapse. The code was developed empirically, eventually allowing the construction of tall, steel-framed structures.

Pursuing this theme, it is instructive to consider the case of steam boilers. In the late eighteenth and throughout the nineteenth centuries English factories were powered by steam engines, the steam being supplied by individual fire-tube boilers. Periodically, there was a boiler explosion, causing deaths and injuries. There were various popular theories as to the cause of these accidents: one being that the operator, in order to obtain more stem pressure, hung a brick on the lever arm of the safety valve. Alternatively, it was supposed that the manufacturer of the boiler, in order to cut costs and increase profits, had made the boiler shell too thin.

In the early twentieth century, following a particularly gruesome boiler accident in a New York laundry, the American Society of Mechanical Engineers set up a committee to write a code for boiler design and construction. Not too long after this event, electric power became available to factories and the boiler problem disappeared. The ASME code, however, has survived and continues to provide invaluable guidance to industry. Also, its use has been made a legal requirement in all the states of the Union, so that, in this instance, the code also serves a political purpose.

After the Second World War it became possible to consider the use of nuclear power for raising steam in central power stations, and the safety of such boilers was a primary concern. Accordingly, investigators in Britain and the USA re-examined records of the early boiler explosions. Both investigations produced the same conclusion: the main cause of the explosions was low water: that is, the boiler had been allowed to boil nearly dry, so the heat of the fire caused pressure to increase until the shell failed and there was an explosion. So, the writing of the ASME boiler code would not have reduced boiler explosion had the situation remained unchanged. It was, nevertheless, a most useful action.

The answer to the original question, therefore, is that it is impossible to predict what effect, if any, the formulation of engineering procedures will have on safety, and they must be justified in their own right. It is probably best to record such developments in the same light as that proposed earlier for technology and science: they contribute to the possibility of improved safety, but whether or not this is achieved, and at what pace, is determined by the human population concerned.

6.3 Mortality from all causes

Plots of mortality rates from all causes against time for different age groups in England and Wales have many features in common, but there are two of special importance. Firstly, they show no evidence of having been affected by doctoring, by the formation of the health service or by the development of effective drugs after the Second World War. And secondly, they are similar in form to plots of accident mortality rates.

During the first three-quarters of the nineteenth century, mortality rates of children and young adults had been declining slowly; then, in about 1870, the plot shows a transition to a sharp purposeful fall. This continued in an irregular fashion for the first half of the twentieth century, by which time the rate had fallen to an irreducibly low level and further development continued at a slow pace. At the same time the general incidence of infectious disease such as typhus, typhoid, dysentery tuberculosis of the lung, etc. showed a corresponding fall. Now this was a time when drugs effective against such diseases had not yet been developed. Thus, this very radical improvement in health was not caused by medication. In Chapter 3 it was ascribed to an acceptance by the population of the germ theory of diseases, such that people began to behave more hygienically, together with the improvements in water quality and sewage disposal.

The plot of mortality rates for older persons in Britain does not show the same early rapid fall; there is a ragged slow decline until the year 1970, after which there was a relatively steep decline with little scatter. This coincides with changes in the records for price inflation and population growth, all of which point to a change towards more cautious behaviour. Figures 6.1 and 6.2 are typical of such plots; they show, respectively, fatality rates due to all causes and to accidents for the male 20–24 and 65–74 age groups.

The pattern of change in mortality rates displayed by such diagrams is best explained as being the result of human behaviour; in particular, the development of skill in avoiding fatal infections. This view is supported by the similarity between all-cause and accident mortality, of which Figs. 6.1 and 6.2 provide an example. It is further reinforced by the figures for the 1918 influenza epidemic, which were analysed in Chapter 3. These showed that the increase in mortality rates due to the epidemic were a maximum for young adults and declined for older people, whilst for those over 65 the

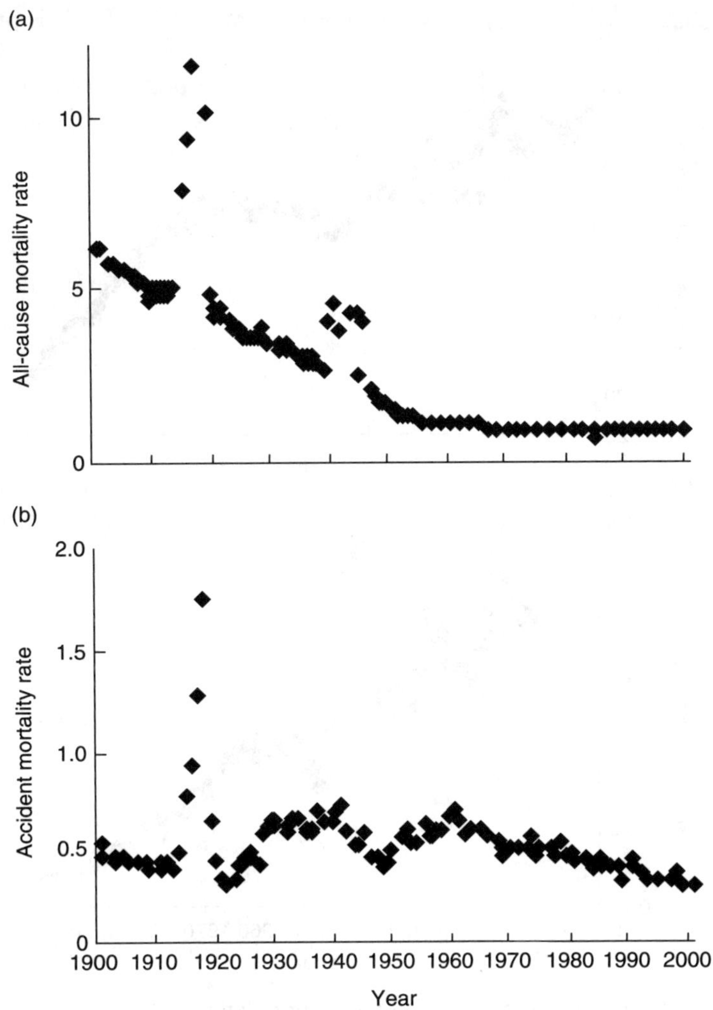

6.1 Annual mortality rate per 1000 population in England and Wales 1901–2000 for the male age group 20–24 (a) from all causes (b) due to accidents. The all-cause mortality rate due to the 1918 influenza epidemic, which was 26, is not shown.

rate even showed a slight fall. It is often asserted that elderly people are most likely to die in an epidemic because of their lower resistance to disease: evidently this is not the case because the probability of infection is the governing factor.

Thus, the rules that apply in the case of fatal accidents are also operative for death from disease. Improvements in medicine and general hygiene make the reduction of mortality rates possible, but the national population

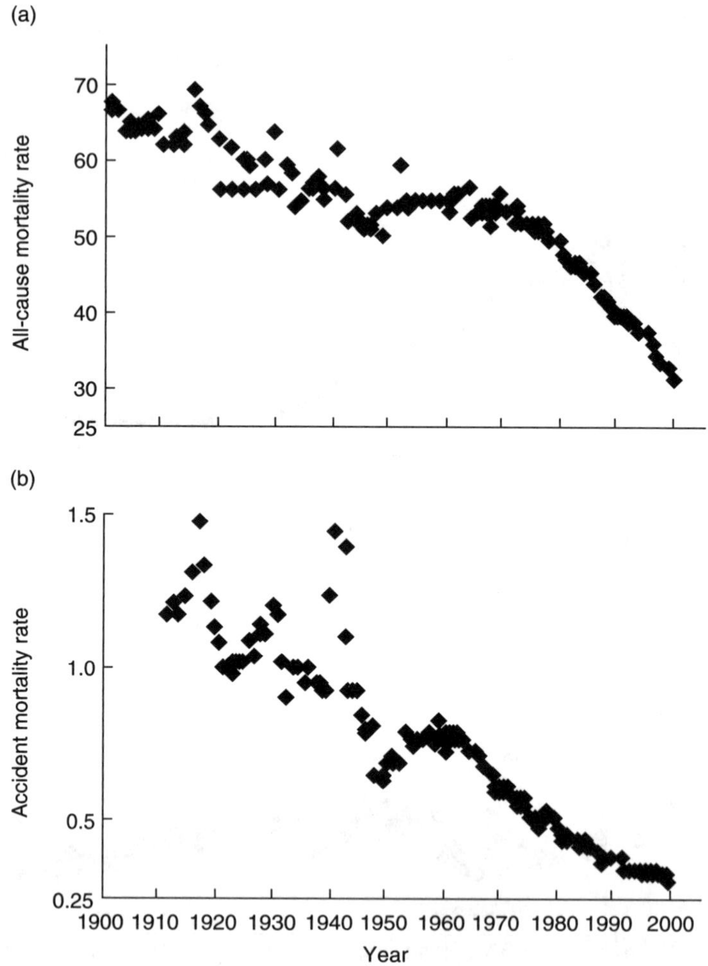

6.2 Annual mortality rate per 1000 population in England and Wales 1901–2000 for the male age group 65–74 (a) from all causes (b) due to accidents.

determines the rate at which this will happen. And, it would seem that death from any cause other than homicide or suicide could reasonably be considered to be a fatal accident.

The role of medicine, according to this doctrine, remains what has always been the case: the relief of suffering for the sick and wounded and their restoration to good health. It is hoped that this task will be accomplished with increasing effectiveness in the future.

6.4 Economic growth

In Chapter 4 it was determined that in Britain, during the second half of the twentieth century, the economic growth rate remained constant during successive periods of different political administrations. Even more significantly, perhaps, there was, in 1979, a change in policy towards a free market, and state-owned companies were sold off to private investors. The efficiency of the industries concerned improved considerably, but the overall growth rate remained the same. Politicians undoubtedly believe that they can manage the economy better than the opposition, so wherein lies the truth?

Now, it is consistent with the general conclusions recorded here that 'the economy', which is the final result of the productive activity of the population as a whole, is regulated, not by a master or a politician, but by itself, and that such regulation is performed subconsciously and collectively. In the nature of things, this results in a gap in comprehension. To the conscious mind, 'the economy' appears to be governed by impersonal forces, and when an economic bubble bursts, we are all, including the politicians, taken by surprise.

So what is to be done? Other than making such adjustments to the rules governing financial and commercial activities that the experience may show to be necessary, there is nothing that it would be possible or desirable to do. It is not possible (fortunately) to direct the behaviour of large populations. And, if politicians wish to believe that they direct the economy of the country, so be it: no great harm will accrue.

It may not be possible for politicians to direct economic growth, but it flourishes best under conditions of political stability. During the first half of the twentieth century, when world politics was in an exceedingly disturbed state, growth in Britain was about 1.5% annually, whilst during the relatively peaceful second half, the annual rise was 2% and, whilst the alternation of political factions in Britain had no effect on growth, the rise of dictatorial regimes that abrogated the rule of law, and the right to own property in Russia and China had a very adverse effect on material prosperity in those countries. It is fortunate that, in the twenty-first century, there is a world-wide trend towards democracy in politics and a free market economy.

6.5 Predictions

It has been a notable feature of the investigations reported in this book that plots of, say, fatal accident rates against time will, on occasion, show a sudden change of direction, and such changes have, quite reasonably, been interpreted as indicating a change of behaviour amongst those people concerned. It would be most useful to a stockbroker to have a test which would indicate the attitude change from hope to fear that precipitates a fall of stock prices, but nobody has yet devised such a test. Thus there is an inherent unpredictability about human affairs such that, no matter how consistent the historical record may be to date, its continuance on the same path cannot be guaranteed. Thus, quantitative history may be very useful in throwing light on areas of human behaviour that would otherwise have remained hidden, but it will not predict the future.

6.6 A negative factor

There is a current belief that could have a damaging effect on economic growth: this stems from the idea that human beings, by burning fossil fuels, have caused an undesirable change in the surface temperature of the earth.

Now economic development requires increasing energy consumption, and this is best supplied by coal and oil. Alternative natural sources are inadequate, and nuclear power sources generate radioactive waste, which would generate a cumulative disposal problem.

The carbon dioxide molecule absorbs energy that is radiated in the visible light range and emits such energy at a longer wavelength: that is, as heat rather than as light. Thus, it has been proposed that the increase in the carbon dioxide constant of the atmosphere due to human activity must result in an increase in the amount of heat radiated towards the Earth, and this is responsible for the observed rise in temperature of the Earth.

Carbon dioxide molecules are a component of a transparent gas mixture, the Earth's atmosphere. Therefore, any radiation will occur in all directions, so that half will be directed towards the Earth, and half away from it. So, the net effect of such a gas on Earth temperatures will be neutral.

This conclusion is supported by empirical observations. When life began on Earth, there was no oxygen in the atmosphere, which consisted mainly of a mixture of nitrogen and carbon dioxide. The oxygen in our present atmosphere has been produced by the action of green plants which, using energy absorbed from solar radiation combine carbon dioxide from the atmosphere with water from the soil to form carbohydrates (initially sugar) and oxygen. In effect, green plants strip the carbon atom out of the carbon dioxide molecule and use it to manufacture the innumerable carbon compounds which constitute living matter. So, the carbon dioxide content of the primeval atmosphere must have been approximately the same as its current oxygen content: about one-fifth.

Now living forms, consisting as they do largely of complex carbon compounds, can only exist within a narrow range of temperatures: more or less those which obtain on Earth today. Thus, Earth surface temperatures with an atmosphere containing 20% CO_2 were more or less the same as those with an atmosphere containing 0.03% CO_2 (this being the CO_2 content at the beginning of the twentieth century). So, the amount of carbon dioxide in the atmosphere has had no significant effect on temperatures at the Earth's surface and the burning of fossil fuels does not have a harmful effect on climate.

Indeed (looking into the distant future), replacing some of the lost carbon dioxide in the atmosphere is beneficial. All animals (including human beings) depend, directly or indirectly, on food that is produced by the photosynthetic reaction in green plants, and this in turn depends on a supply of carbon dioxide from the atmosphere. Now, at a content of 0.03% (probably 0.04% early in the twenty-first century), it is nearly all used up, and there would inevitably have come a time when green plants, and their dependants, the animals, could no longer survive. For better or worse, this particular threat to the continuance of life on earth, has been averted.

In past millennia, there have been many variations in the Earth's surface temperature, and the present warming phase is in no way unusual. Any theory that claims to account for such warming must also account for the Ice Ages, and this the CO_2 theory cannot do. There is, however, one possibility that is worth considering: namely, that the Earth is itself a heat source, and that the surface temperature generated by this source is variable.

The Earth contains a small proportion of radioactive elements, principally uranium. These elements generate heat, such that there is a temperature gradient from the centre outwards. The surface temperature is determined by the balance between heat absorbed from solar radiation, plus that conducted and convected from the interior, and heat radiated from the surface into space.

Now the movement of tectonic plates (that which gives rise to earthquakes) and of continents provides evidence for convectional flow in the mantle (that is, the region between the molten core and the surface crust of the Earth). The mantle is composed of solid material, and it is supposed that this behaves like a fluid of very high viscosity – as does ice, when flowing under the influence of gravity in a glacier. Now, radioactive elements are not uniformly distributed within the Earth, but are present as discrete deposits. When these are more numerous near the surface, there will be a warm phase, and when they are more numerous near the core, there will be an Ice Age. Such underground heating would be expected to result in warmer winters and higher night time temperatures, but would not significantly affect daytime or summer maxima. Such appears to be the case in Southern England.

6.7 Final comments

This chapter started with a series of questions which arose from the conclusion that human affairs are regulated subconsciously and collectively by the relevant population. This being so, it was asked, what is the point in devising regulations that are intended to reduce accident and all-cause mortality and control economic growth? These matters were discussed in some detail, but the short answer to this question is that, whilst such actions may, fortuitously, be beneficial, they have no effect on the mortality or economic growth rates. More generally: political instability, and, in particular the two World Wars of the twentieth century, caused perturbations, but did not significantly affect the trend of these various rates.

In Britain, fatal accident rates fell during the period for which records are available: that is, from 1858 onwards. This fall is ascribed to the development of skill on the part of the national population, such that people became more adept in avoiding mishaps. This progress was made possible by technological change, which made transport and industry safer, and led to considerable improvements in domestic conditions.

The human behaviour associated with the reduction of accident mortality rates was one of caution, while those concerned were not consciously aware of this, or the process whereby safety was improved. This process was, it must be concluded, subconsciously and collectively regulated.

Most fatal accidents occur to males. At birth, both sexes are equal in this respect but, with increasing age, they diverge to a maximum at ages between 20 and 30, when the ratio between male and female accident mortality rates is in the range 5 to 10. With increasing age, the ratio falls, typically to about 2. Thus, fatal accident rates are also biologically regulated; this fact lends force to the conclusion that the reduction of fatal accident rate with time is subconsciously regulated.

Plots of mortality rates from all causes versus time for the various male age groups are remarkably similar to those for male accident fatality rates. In both cases there is a general decrease during the twentieth century. For youths and young men there is a similar upsurge corresponding to the two World Wars, and for older men a similar linear fall during the period 1970–2000. If it is assumed that the dominant factor amongst those which govern the all-cause mortality rate is the risk of infection by a fatal disorder, then this similarity makes sense. Thus, the general fall in mortality rates results from more hygienic behaviour – that is greater skill in avoiding infection, together with improved water supply and sewage disposal. The upsurge during the two World Wars resulted from a higher acceptance of risk by young men, and the downturn in 1970 was associated with more cautious behaviour generally. Indeed, mortality in general may be regarded as the result of a fatal accident.

However this may be, the rules that were developed for fatal accidents also applied to the mortality from all causes, and in particular, mortality rates and longevity are regulated by the national population, and not by doctors.

The ratio between male and female mortality from all causes follows a similar trend to that for accidents, being greatest for young adults, but the difference between the sexes is less.

The fear of death provides a very strong incentive for the reduction of mortality rates, and instances where fatality rates increase with time are exceptional and usually short-lived. No such limitation is in place for the economy, and no matter where growth occurs, whether of prices generally, house prices, share prices or national output, there is a tendency for the rise to accelerate to a point of instability, followed by a sudden collapse. Such economic slumps occur as perturbations of an exponential rise in national output; they are uncomfortable at the time, but probably serve a useful purpose in weeding out inefficient organisations. There is a general inverse relationship between economic growth and the fall in mortality rates, also there was, in Britain, a more direct connection in the period 1970–2000, when price inflation changed from an exponential to a linear rise, whilst at the same time accident and all-cause mortality rates for older people changed to a steep linear fall.

Overall, therefore, historical records in Britain are consistent with the view that the increase of prosperity, safety and longevity results from a development of skill by the national population, and that this development is subconsciously and collectively regulated. Britain is not unique as a country, and it must be supposed that the same characteristics apply to other developing nations.

6.8 The world turned upside-down

It is appropriate, therefore, to re-phrase earlier questions and ask: if safety, health and prosperity are regulated by the national population, what should be the function of government, and of agencies that have responsibility for safety and health?

The first answer to this question must be that, whatever the function, the attitude of such bodies should be one of humility; the recognition that they should exist as servants and not as masters. There has indeed been a trend in this direction: from the Pharaohs of ancient Egypt, who were revered as gods, through Charles I of England, who considered himself to be God's viceroy, to the twentieth-century Scandinavian king who travelled to the office on a bicycle. On the other hand, there is an increasing tendency by safety zealots to devise both caps that cannot be removed and cans that will not open, and to ban useful substances less they be eaten by a two-year-old child. There is much to be said for the study of accident mortality records to obtain a balanced view on how best to assure safety.

6.9 Safety policy

One final question: bearing in mind the results of this study, what action should be taken to minimise the risk of fatal accidents?

The first step, in answer to this question, is to recognise that the cause-and-effect theory of fatal accidents is fundamentally unsound. According to this theory (which is unstated but whose precepts are widely accepted), all accidents have a cause, and by identifying and eliminating these causes, accident mortality can be reduced. The basic defect of this theory is that it treats the human being as a cipher, devoid of understanding or volition. In fact, human beings are intelligent and have a lively desire for self-preservation. And, the observed fall of fatal accident rates with time is consistent with the view that the human factor is dominant. Seeking out all possible causes of risk and designing against them leads to over-elaborate equipment that is likely to be unreliable in service. The best designs, from all points of view, are those that produce devices that are uncomplicated and easy to use.

It has been established here (and in the book by Duffey and Small – see Appendix) that, in most of the human activities examined, fatality rates due to accidents are falling. Such falls are regulated subconsciously, but are made possible by advances in science and technology. Thus, conscious efforts to improve safety are best directed towards technological development, for example, making vehicles easier to drive and stronger, and improving the road system. It must be accepted, however, that there is no direct connection between the two spheres of activity, and the pace of fatality reduction will not immediately reflect the pattern of technological change.

There remain those instances where fatality rates are not falling in a regulated fashion – for example, motorcycling and some activities in the oil industry. Motorcycling is a sport whose attraction is, to a substantial degree, the fact that it is hazardous. There is no established technique for altering human behaviour in such cases, but the general fall in the level of acceptable risk amongst young men may well bring about an improvement.

Since accident mortality rates in Britain are falling in a regulated manner and at a satisfactory rate, there is no case for governmental intervention. In matters that concern safety, governmental agencies should restrict their activities to the collection, monitoring and dissemination of data, and should not attempt to make rules for a situation that is already adequately controlled.

Appendix: Sources

It is the custom in scientific and technical publications to provide numbered references to individual papers or books that provide supporting evidence. In the present work, however, the sources are numerical lists derived from annual publications of governmental and other agencies, and to set these out for each chapter would have been repetitive. These sources are, therefore, listed below under subject headings.

Mortality rates during the nineteenth century in England and Wales

Table entitled 'Causes of death' in the Registrar-General's: *Annual Statistical Review* (published annually 1838–1974).

'Population, England and Wales, 1801–2001'. Table supplied by Office for National Statistics, London.

Gives population according to age group and sex at 10-year intervals.

All-cause and accident mortality, twentieth century

Twentieth Century Mortality compact disc issue by the Office for National Statistics, London.

Gives annual number of deaths according to age group and sex against the cause as listed in the International Classification of Disease, which includes accidents, and which is also listed. Includes relevant population figures. All data are for England and Wales.

Fatality rates in transport and industry

Air transport

Statistical Summary of Commercial Jet Aircraft Accidents Boeing Commercial Aircraft Group, Seattle USA (published annually).

British manufacturing industry

Numbers of Persons Killed in Industrial Accidents, 1860 to 1968 Historical Injury Data, Health and Safety Executive, London.

British Labour Statistics Department of Employment 1971, H.M. Stationery Office, London.

Fatal Injury Rates, 1981 to 2000 Health and Safety Executive, London.

Economic growth

Feinstein, C.H. *National Income, Expenditure and Output of the United Kingdom, 1855 to 1965* Cambridge University Press, 1972.

Data supplied by the Office for National Statistics, London.

Financial loss due to accidents on oil refineries

Large Property Damage Losses in the Hydrocarbon-Chemical Industry 20th Edition 2003, Marsh and McLennan, Chicago, USA.

Natural disasters

World Disasters The International Federation of Red Cross and Red Crescent Societies (published annually).

Rail transport

Data furnished by the Railway Inspectorate, The Health and Safety Executive, London.

Offshore operations

World Offshore Accidental Databank Det Norske Veritas, Oslo, Norway published annually 1964–1997. Post-1997 data held by Det Norske Veritas.

Road transport

Road Accidents Great Britain Office for National Statistics, London (published annually).

World Disasters 1988 The International Federation of Red Cross and Red Crescent Societies, London.

Sea transport

Lloyd's Casualty Report Annual Statistical Summary Lloyd's Register of Shipping, London.

Previous work

As observed in the text, the subject matter of this book does not fall within the scope of any contemporary academic discipline, and there is no coherent body of research to which reference can be made. The correlation between road accident fatality rates and national prosperity was noted by R.J. Smead, an account of whose work is given by J. Adams in the *Proceedings of the General Motors 1968 Conference on Human Behaviour and Traffic Safety*. R.B. Duffey and J.W. Saull analyse accident mortality data in the book *Know the Risk* and find that such rates decline with the passage of time.

An outline of the present book will be found in

Lancaster, J: *Engineering Catastrophes* 3rd edn, Woodhead Publishing Limited and CRC Press, 2005.

The effect of radioactive elements on earth temperatures is discussed in *Conduction of Heat in Solids* by H.S. Carslaw and J.C. Jaeger, Clarendon Press, Oxford.

Index